The journey is the reward.

Tao saying

Awakening the
TIGER
Within

9 PATHS TO HEALING AND EMPOWERMENT

Joy Heartsong

MS, CHTP

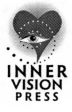

INNER
VISION
PRESS

Awakening the Tiger Within
9 Paths to Healing and Empowerment
By Joy Heartsong, MS, CHTP

NOTE: Client stories are factual. The names have been changed to protect their privacy.

Editor: Kim Pearson, www.primary-sources.com
Copyeditor: Christine Frank, www.christinefrank.com
Index: Christine Frank, www.christinefrank.com
Cover and Interior design: Dawn Putney and Toolbox Creative, www. toolboxcreative.com
Photograph of the Author: Jodi Lewis, www.jodistyle.com

Library of Congress Cataloguing-in-Publications Data
Library of Congress Control Number: 2007937588
Joy Heartsong
Awakening the Tiger Within: 9 Paths to Healing and Empowerment
ISBN: 978-0-9799818-0-7
Library of Congress subject headings:
1. Healing   2. Self-help   3. Body, Mind & Spirit
2007

Table of Contents

APPENDIX

Taking Your Tiger by the Tail

Acknowledgements

My friends, family, and clients are, without a doubt, almost as delighted as I am to see this book manifested into form. For many months they have watched it grow from a seed of an idea to a living, breathing expression of vital energy. This transformation has come into being through a very supportive, creative team of individuals and the guidance of Spirit and the inner tiger.

I give thanks for my three wonderful children, Mark, Paul, and Jennifer, and families, who are confidently exploring their own paths. I appreciate their interest, support, and ideas.

To Jack Mallicoat, gentle, strong tiger, I am grateful for your patience, willingness to listen and offer input, and for always being there for me. Your encouragement is a constant source of motivation and strength.

My gratitude also goes to all the women who guided me and taught me what it takes to birth a book.

First, a big "thank you, thank you" goes to my friends in our writing group. To Marsha Rand, I appreciate you and your wealth of experience, your unending flow of great ideas, and your positive approach to everything. To Mary Jane Gilson, I am grateful for your loving support, your candid feedback, and the constructive suggestions you've offered. To Lisa McElvaney, sweet, gentle heart, for your wisdom in both the physical and non-physical realms and for encouraging me to share more of my personal story at a deeper level.

Thank you all for the plethora of creative ideas, the depth of your knowing, and your unwavering faith in me and my ability to share from my heart and my experience. All three of you are fabulous examples of women who go with the flow and make life look easy and peaceful while moving through the challenges life presents.

To my friend Linda Bosserman, thank you for the many, many invaluable hours of listening, sharing, and computer support. What a blessing you are!

To Jan King, Founder and Editorial Director of the eWomenPublishing Network, I want to give thanks for your kind, encouraging manner and words, for your positive feedback, and for the fabulous training and mentoring you provided.

My gratitude goes to Gail Richards, creative founder of Author Smart, who provided extensive support by making numerous resources for training and tracking the book writing and publishing process so readily available. The teleconferences and Brown Bag Lunch conference calls have been both practical and inspiring.

Finally, I wish to acknowledge and thank my wonderful clients for their stories, encouragement, and desire to explore healing and wholeness at deeper levels. The trust they have placed in me has encouraged me to explore the inner depths of energy healing with them.

WELCOME TO AWAKENING A NEW YOU—a new way of seeing yourself and the world around you. We come into this world with the desire and ability to fully use our power. However, most of us cloud or forget this truth very early in life. Therefore, we seek that faint memory of the tiger within: the power that lies deep inside each of us.

Since ancient times and throughout a variety of cultures, the tiger has been looked upon as a symbol of courage, bravery, and strength, and has been associated with yang (male energy). The tiger also represents the power that connects directly with Spirit, the higher power, and inner wisdom, the yin (female energy). As such, it is a perfect symbol of empowerment, blending courage with inner strength and wisdom.

You are about to embark on an exciting journey of self-healing and empowerment. This book will help increase your awareness, your belief in yourself, and your ability to listen to and follow your inner wisdom. You will feel more joy and peace in your life.

About the Words

When we plan a trip, it is helpful to know the language of the land or culture we will be visiting. In some cases, we may already speak the language of the people. In other cases, we may plan to use an interpreter or a conversational guidebook.

For our journey together, I have defined some common words in a way that may seem somewhat uncommon to you. The usage of the words below relates to healing and empowerment.

Abundance is a belief that we are immersed in unlimited potential, creative possibilities, and timelessness rather than striving for all the worldly things we want when we want them.

'All That Is' is another way of referring to God, Spirit, or a higher power.

Joy is more than just happiness. Happiness relates to the temporary emotional state in the world of people, things, and occurrences. Joy describes a higher energetic frequency; joy is the eternal state of being in harmony with all that is.

Love is eternal, sacred, and unconditional. It is the language of Spirit, All That Is, God, and an open heart. Love is feeling oneness with all that is.

Peace is a state of inner calm and allowing what is.

Spirit is synonymous with God, Buddha, Mohammed, Jehovah, All That Is, Creator, Infinite Wisdom, or any of the names used by people throughout the world for a higher power. Please substitute whatever name you prefer.

Now that we know we're speaking the same language, let's continue on.

I wrote this book to share my experience, my training, and my heart to facilitate your healing process. As the book gently unfolded, it showed me what is deep inside in the personal process of healing from within. My wonderful, awakening clients shared some of their journeys, insights, dreams, and experiences that you may identify with, learn from, and take courage from.

Very recently, with the help of a friend, I realized the root of my passion for helping others learn to use their power began in childhood, observing and interacting with my grandparents and parents. While I had glimpses of an inner power or inner guidance in my earlier years, these moments were all too fleeting. Much of the time they seemed entirely beyond my grasp.

I know first-hand the challenges we face in staying hopeful, loving, and peaceful when surrounded by people who are not. As a child, I experienced both abuse and abandonment. I was shy, lonely, unhappy, and reluctant to speak up or speak out. As an adult, emotional abuse, life-threatening illness, and loss were critical parts of my life.

There is nothing particularly remarkable about my personal journey. Now I know that it just is. Now I know we shape our experiences. We attract people, situations, and things to us by our thoughts and feelings. *(Sometimes)*

Are you feeling mired down, in a rut, bored, frustrated, hopeless, or helpless? The great temptation is to blame others or the circumstances in which we find ourselves. Surely we can point the finger for our fear, our unhappiness, our lack of progress, or our "stuckness" at someone else...or can we?

We can learn to love life even when things are not going the way we envisioned. If we're not happy or peaceful with ourselves or with our life situation, we can change it. I have that power, and so do you.

This is the message you will hear over and over in this book: You have always had the power of the tiger. You can never truly lose it. You can, however, learn to use it more effectively to create the life of your heart's desire. I am passionate about helping you know this truth, helping you believe it, and helping you claim your power.

Each of us has a tiger deep within, whether we recognize it or not, that guides us on our healing journey. Are you aware of yours? In this book, you will learn how to listen to and follow it.

> We can learn to love life even when things are not going the way we envisioned.

Now is the time to connect with your inner power and learn how to use it. Now is the time to start communicating your feelings and your boundaries. Now is the time to enjoy your freedom and begin living the life of your heart's desire.

This book is for you if you are:

- Searching for something more than what you have
- Seeking a deeper meaning or purpose in life, committed to making changes in your life
- Prepared to face your fears and take action to move beyond them
- Developing an openness to other ways of thinking and being
- Focused on reclaiming your power and seeking help using it
- Willing to change how you feel about yourself and your life
- Healing and looking for support in this process
- Beginning to listen to your body, guidance and intuition and wishing to develop that ability more fully
- Desiring more peace, love, joy and abundance in your life

Awakening the Tiger Within addresses the use of inner power and ways of discovering how to use it as a path to inner peace. You will read stories from my work with clients, from personal experiences, and from connections with other people that illustrate the nine paths to healing and empowerment. Empowerment guides, action guides, and healing guides are included at the end of each chapter. They contain a wide variety of techniques, suggestions, and inspirational tips to aid in your journey of self-healing.

Think of this journey as you would an adventure to a new land with a different culture and language. Be open to new ideas, experiences, and ways of communicating. See how the new words feel to your tongue. Taste the food and drink. Form new relationships with yourself and others.

Awakening the Tiger Within is like a travel guide that takes you on new journeys to a familiar place or to uncharted lands. Come and explore the nine paths on the journey with me. You may choose to pursue one or all of them. Find the one that connects you most completely with that stillness deep inside.

Any path can help you awaken the tiger and lead to healing. You get to choose. Listen, follow, and allow what is.

Move beyond the fear that has kept you from being peaceful and joyful. Find out how to take pleasure in each day, excited to be doing what you are guided to do. Explore techniques used by clients, both men and women, which have helped them turn their lives around and move beyond their blocks and fears. Discover joy in the simple things in life as well as those you consider more significant or purposeful.

From this guided experience, take what resonates with you. Leave behind what doesn't. Make a commitment to see yourself, your life, and "all that is" differently. Share this journey with others who are also seeking something more than what they are currently experiencing.

Keep in mind...it's not about being better, smarter, richer, or faster. It's not about changing yourself into something grander, holier, or more deserving. It *is* about being willing to learn to connect with and trust your inner power and use it.

Now let's take the next step on the journey of healing and empowerment by turning the page and looking at some of our fears and limiting beliefs and how they can sap our power.

We keep our
tiger confined
in a very tiny cage
when we let
fear control our
choices.

CHAPTER ONE

The **Tiger** and the **Cage**

Releasing Fears and Limiting Beliefs

THE PAST HAS NO POWER OVER YOU except what you give it.

Fear is the number one obstacle to empowerment and love. If we're feeling fear, we're not feeling love. We cannot feel opposite emotions in the same exact moment. Therefore, the more fearful we are, the less time we're spending in love. Releasing fears and limiting beliefs is the first path to healing and empowerment.

Fill in these blanks. "I can't do that because I'm _____ someone will think I'm crazy (or will laugh at me)... I'm not going to get involved in another relationship because I'm _____ I'll get hurt again ...If I do that, I'm _____ I'll lose my job."

Most of you probably filled in the blank with the same word: afraid. Fear comes up so easily and frequently in our daily living that we often don't recognize how much it influences our thinking and behaviors.

Fear keeps us locked into a paradigm that says, "If you're not vigilant, the world (or someone in it) will hurt you. Be careful! Look out! What you don't know may harm you. Remember your past!"

Fear binds us to this world of form and saps our energy. We keep our tiger confined in a very tiny cage when we let fear control our choices.

Are you buying into a lifestyle based on fear? Maybe you feel there's not enough to go around. Or you're afraid you don't really deserve the good things in life. Maybe you feel you don't have the power to make a difference; that you have to resign yourself to being sick, lonely, over-worked, or stressed instead of doing what you'd really like to do.

Is this a pattern you've developed? Take a look at your habitual thoughts. For example: *"I'll never be able to do that…My father won't like it…I'm afraid that…"* Then ask yourself how your thoughts make you feel, both physically and emotionally.

Have you ever found yourself saying any of these: "Oh, I could never do that! What will my mother (father, friends, spouse) say?...I'm afraid that _____." Look at the fear-based statements that come to you. Discern where they came from and how you can begin shifting some of them.

You may have developed a pattern that keeps you from doing or saying what you'd really like to do. Think about how you feel physically and emotionally when you respond like this.

Others may try to discourage you by saying: "You're crazy if you think _____ will happen. You're not really going to do that, are you?"

Then there's the "poor me" attitude: "What am *I* supposed to do? How do you think *I* feel?"

You may respond by saying, "You're probably right," and then change your plan. You may get angry and defensive, and then change your plan. You may get upset with the people who challenge you, and then give up. Or perhaps you continue with your course of action and feel good about yourself.

So often we let voices from our ego self and others convince us not to follow what we *know* is best. We let fears keep us from moving forward into new ways of seeing and being. We're usually unaware of how much fear controls our choices and our lives.

You may hang onto old beliefs that no longer serve who you are or have become. You may use the old beliefs out of habit or fear, or from not examining the source of the belief. Ask yourself, "Is that really true, or have I just convinced myself that it is?"

We are usually very strongly influenced by what others think and do. It's a lot like looking in a mirror. Often you may frown and think, "I'm not happy with that person." Then you go about your day feeling unhappy and dissatisfied. Sometimes you may like what you see. Then you smile and feel good about yourself all day.

On a spiritual level, other people are like reflecting mirrors. If they express impatience with you, or seem to be unreliable, critical, negative, lazy, or dishonest, you may become upset with them. Then you may also feel bad about yourself, your work, and your relationships. If they compliment you, smile at you, and support you, you smile and feel better.

"What others think of me is none of my business."

If you wake up feeling good about yourself and your life in general, you may feel terrible right after your first interaction with a challenging situation or a critical person. When this happens, closely examine what occurred to bring about that shift in your attitude. You'll often find that you reacted negatively because the encounter *triggered* something deep inside you.

When we're sensitive to something or are trying to deny it, we're more defensive. Perhaps the other person's behavior reminds you of your unsupportive father. The situation may bring back your feelings of not being "enough" in some way. So you either lash out or internalize it. Then you feel bad about yourself. Looking into these *mirrors* deeply and honestly can provide great insight and facilitate healing within us.

You may have heard the expression, "What others think of me is none of my business." Great wisdom is inherent in these few words. Do you let your concerns and fears of what others may think influence your thoughts and behaviors? Where you go, whom you associate with, what you wear, and how you spend your money are usually heavily influenced by your experiences and perceptions of how others view you. When you act and think independently of what others think, you are wiser and more in your power than you may realize.

Now let's look at some examples of limiting beliefs.

Joy's Story
Long and Hard

To become certified as a Healing Touch Practitioner, I was required to write a case study and bind it into a booklet along with all of my readings, experiences, and plans. Doing the actual work was fun, fulfilling, and fruitful. However, the writing portion paralyzed me.

Faced with recording and summarizing all I had done during the past year, I felt bogged down, blocked, and beset by doubts. I didn't know where or how to begin this last, "formidable" piece. It was going to be hard and take a long time. I convinced myself I could not get everything completed and submitted by the due date. *Too much to do and too little time* seemed to be my daily mantra. I worried a lot and worked very little.

So I talked to a professional life coach about my lack of progress, my fears, and my concerns. She pointed out how I was self-sabotaging, and together we formulated an affirmation: "Doing this work is going to be fun and easy and will be completed by the due date."

In less than one week of focusing daily on this affirmation, I felt a shift in my attitude, beliefs, and motivation. I started working on what I considered to be the easiest part of the writing and then moved to the next easiest. Before long, nothing seemed difficult. I was actually having fun watching the project come together. And as an added bonus, I put the booklets and the application in the mail one week early.

My belief that this project was going to be difficult and take a long time had been keeping me from making much progress. Not progressing further had reinforced those beliefs. However, what I had previously considered nearly impossible and very distasteful became a pleasant, rewarding, relatively easy task.

Rhonda's Story

Another story of a limiting belief comes from working with a client. I was doing Healing Touch and other energy work with Rhonda when I paused, resting my hand on her thigh. She said with enthusiasm: "You found it! That's where the lock has been for so many years. No one has been able to remove it."

It took a moment to realize that Rhonda was talking about an etheric, unseen lock rather than a physical one. She sensed it both intuitively and from the way the energy felt. Rhonda believed she was unable to make any progress with her work. Something, which she saw as a lock, was restricting her freedom to move forward.

Now I felt it too and connected with it intuitively. I laughed and told her the lock was rusty. "It's been there a long time. It needs to be oiled before it can be released." I applied Release, a therapeutic-grade essential oil blend to her leg.

I got another message for Rhonda amid much laughter: "Guess what? It's not even locked! And...furthermore, you're the one who put it there, so you must be the one to remove it."

I encouraged Rhonda to release the lock when she was ready. She immediately reached down to her leg and removed it. Rhonda said she could feel the energy releasing in her leg. She expressed her gratitude for being free of the lock.

Can you see ways you may have metaphorically placed a lock on yourself? Most of us hold ourselves back in some way. We often act from *shoulds* rather than from *knowing* what we really want to do. We let our fears override our intuition much of the time. Our perception of our limitations and abilities keep us from moving forward with our desires or our guidance.

We blame our circumstances, health, other people, physical abilities, or attributes for our unhappiness, anger, or perceived lack of worldly "success." A popular refrain is, "I had a really horrible childhood. I was poor, abused, neglected, unloved ..." Other excuses might include: "My husband doesn't want me to." "My mother won't like it." "My boss is a tyrant."

Surely you've heard these stories or explanations for where someone is in life or for feeling the way someone does. Even you may have used a similar story to explain your life situation.

Another common lament is, "If only I had (or hadn't) _____." You can complete this from your experience. Here are some that may sound familiar. "If only I hadn't fallen asleep at the wheel...If only I had looked into it closer before I invested my life savings (crossed the street, took the job)...If only I hadn't let him persuade me to give him one more chance."

The list goes on and on. "I'm a loser...I don't believe (can't trust, can't see how) _____." Limiting beliefs about others or ourselves keep us from moving forward. We often get stuck on how things should be or the "right" way to do things. When we do, these beliefs act as locks and blocks to peace and the inner flow of abundance and joy.

In these examples, power is given to the past, other people, or a life situation. This is always a losing position. You may know someone who is feeling trapped by his fears and beliefs. You may be using the past as a reason for not being happy in this moment. If so, you've given your power away. As a result, you have little left to use in your present circumstances. You may feel stuck, defeated, hopeless, and depressed. In short, you feel victimized and see no way out, even when others offer encouragement and help.

"So," you may be saying, "now that I see some ways I give away my power, what can I do to reclaim it?" One of the most basic things you can do for yourself is to change your perception of yourself and the world around you. We'll come back to this later in this chapter with some specific ways to do this.

Jodi's Story

First, here's a story of a woman who turned a limiting belief into empowerment. A few years ago I met a woman named Jodi in a class I was teaching called "Healing Yourself with Healing Touch." I explained the energy field or aura around the body as well as some of the primary chakras or energy centers affecting the flow of energy in the body. I guided the students to practice feeling their energy and use some Healing Touch techniques.

Jodi said, "I can't feel the energy. How come I can't when everyone else can? What's wrong with me?"

I responded with, "It's okay if you don't feel the energy. Just do the work anyway and imagine that it's balancing and clearing the energy. The techniques are effective even if you can't feel anything. As you do the work more and more, you'll start feeling the energy." At that point, I didn't sense I had reassured Jodi or convinced her of anything.

About one week after the class, Jodi called me and, in a very animated voice, shared the following story.

Jodi started with, "I healed myself!"

"Wonderful," I responded. "How did you do that?"

Jodi explained. "I went to the fitness club to work out. However, I had a pain in my back and couldn't do anything without pain. Then I remembered what you taught us. I put my hand on my back to see if I could release the pain. Guess what? It actually went away. I could hardly believe it!"

I congratulated Jodi and encouraged her to continue using the techniques. I thanked her for calling to share her experience with me.

Clearly, a shift had taken place in Jodi. She began as a student in an introductory Healing Touch class who believed she couldn't be an effective healer because she didn't feel the energy. However, Jodi used the techniques, and, even though she still didn't feel the energy, she felt the result: pain relief.

Jodi changed her perception of her own ability to heal. She also was willing to let go of an old belief. These shifts moved her from a feeling of powerlessness to one of empowerment. Kudos go to Jodi for pushing through her limiting belief and doing it anyway.

The limiting belief takes the form of, "I can't do this because _____." The blank in this case can be filled with: *I'm not good enough, smart enough, or talented enough*. This often leads to another limiting belief as it did with Jodi: "There must be something wrong with me." At this point, many people give up and won't try again. They feel powerless to succeed.

It can be challenging to let go of fears and limiting beliefs. However, it is possible to move beyond them and not let them keep you from changing your life. The past is gone. It has no power over you except what you give it. *(Not entirely true)*

Seven Steps to Reclaim Your Power

Here are seven basic steps to reclaiming the power you may have given away to fear and limiting beliefs.

1. The first step is increasing your awareness of your fears and limiting beliefs. Notice how they affect your behaviors, responses, and interactions and how they control you. Start making a list of those areas that come into your awareness.

2. Have you decided that you're ready to change? Desire is a powerful motivator. This is the second step.

3. The third step is willingness and commitment to work at making changes. You may desire change, but if you're not going to do anything differently, change is not very likely to occur. Once you really are willing to change, a higher power or your spiritual guides will help you with this.

4. The fourth step is to focus on one fear or limiting belief you want to change. You may choose the one that seems the easiest

to you, or the least intimidating. Perhaps you want to work on one that feels most restrictive to you or makes you the most unhappy or annoyed. You may just get a feeling for which one is right for you to start with. Write it down.

5. Visualizing yourself making the change you desire is the fifth step. Do it several times a day. It's also important to feel the emotions that accompany that shift.

6. The sixth step is to plan specific ways to change your old pattern or release the fear. *Feel the fear and do it anyway* is a mantra some people choose to live by. Another way to think of it is: *Don't worry that you can't fly. Jump and grow your wings on the way down.* Really!?

   You may decide to set and enforce your boundaries with other people, say affirmations, pray, or make a power state-ment. You may find it easiest to start with a very small change. Write it down. Read it every morning and every evening. Now begin implementing your plan. Focus on it, take steps toward it, and feel good about it daily.

   Think of moving through fear as being a little like learning to walk. You take one small step, steady yourself from your new position, and take another step. Then you take two more steps with greater confidence and trust in yourself. If you temporarily lose your balance and fall, get up and keep going.

7. The last step is to reward yourself for the changes you're making. You can celebrate by having a party, treating yourself to something special, patting yourself on the back, or just smiling and feeling good all over. You can share your successes with a supportive friend or spouse or write them down and review them from time to time.

It takes desire to see things differently and/or total surrender, letting go of your beliefs about how things should be. "I could see peace instead of this," from *A Course in Miracles* can be a life-changing message. Change your mind and you change your world. Does it feel like your tiger's locked in a cage or roaming free?

Empowerment Guide

- Feeling afraid is a condition of being human. Nearly everyone is afraid of something. How you deal with your fears determines whether you are losing your power or using it.

- Feeling healed and empowered requires moving beyond fear and negativity.

- While you may like to blame others or your life situation for your "stuckness" or lack, it's your own fears and beliefs that keep you trapped where you are.

- Using the past as an excuse for your present condition is a power drainer and serves no useful purpose.

- To facilitate change, you must be willing to change something. Believe that change is normal and desirable.

- The seven steps to releasing fears and limiting beliefs are:

  1. Increase awareness of your fears and beliefs.
  2. Desire and be open to change.
  3. Be willing and committed to working on releasing old patterns.
  4. Focus on letting go of one fear or limiting belief at a time.
  5. Visualize and feel the change you desire.
  6. Plan and implement the changes.
  7. Reward yourself for your progress.

Action Guide

Affirmations:

Write and say your own affirmation based on the model earlier in this chapter or on the one below. Use the limiting beliefs you have, and change them into a positive form. Be sure it's what you truly desire.

Even though I feel some fear about _____, I am doing it anyway.

Energy Technique:

When a fear comes up for you, recline in a comfortable place or sit in a relaxed position as soon as possible. Close your eyes and focus your attention on your body. Notice where you feel stress, tightness, or tension. Hold one or both hands on this area(s).

Does it feel like your tiger's locked in a cage or roaming free?

Now start breathing as though you're breathing in and out of that area. (It may be your abdomen, solar plexus, heart, neck, or shoulders, or another place.) Breathe in through your nose and out through your mouth. Increase your awareness of how that part of your body feels. You may experience warmth or cold. You may have a sense of feeling stuck, sad, angry, or afraid. Colors, words, or flashbacks from another time may come to you.

Allow whatever you're sensing to be as it is without trying to judge, control, or stifle it. After you connect deeply with this part of your body, begin to focus on allowing the tight, congested energy and stress to begin releasing. Continue until you feel calmer, lighter, or more peaceful. While still holding your hands on your body and breathing in the same way, visualize that area filling with a peaceful blue light. (You may choose to use a different color if you are drawn to another one.) When it feels complete to you, you're ready to gently bring your focus back to your hands, your feet, and the space around you.

Inner Connecting: Tiger Freedom

Sit or lie quietly. Take five deep breaths. With each breath, relax your muscles and release anything that doesn't feel calm and peaceful. With each exhale, let go of any stress, tension, anger, fear, or hate.

Now focus your attention on your kidneys, located at your low back just above the waist. The kidneys are associated primarily with fear. Notice how the energy at your kidneys feels. Imagine you can breathe in and out of your kidneys. Notice anything else that may come to your attention. When you are feeling more love or you have focused on the kidneys for a couple minutes, shift your focus to the liver, located below your ribs on the right side.

The liver is the organ usually connected with anger. Start breathing as though you can breathe in and out of your liver. Notice any feelings or thoughts that may come up for you. Just allow them to be and continue focusing your attention at your liver. Be willing to release any anger that you may feel in this area. Keep your attention on your liver for several minutes. As this area feels calmer, shift your focus to your throat.

Your throat stores congested energy related to communication and speaking your truth. Breathe in and out of your throat, becoming aware of anything that comes up for you here. Be willing to release any stuck energy and old patterns related to communicating your truth. Feel it gently and completely letting go...Now begin breathing peace and confidence into your throat. Continue allowing that wonderful energy to fill your throat.

Next, move your attention to your third eye, located at your brow above the nose. Focus your attention here, feeling the energy expanding and becoming lighter and freer. Visualize a more open, connected feeling with your inner self, the tiger within.

When you feel peaceful energy filling and surrounding your being, bring your attention back to your body and the space around you. Move your fingers and toes. Open your eyes and have a joy-filled day.

Essential Oils:

Patchouly (Patchouli), Sandalwood, and Melissa

- Patchouly has a sedating, calming, relaxing effect and helps reduce anxiety. Use it in a diffuser or apply to the bottom of your feet.

- Sandalwood helps you accept others, decrease negative feelings, and balance emotions. Apply it to your feet or third eye at your brow just above the nose.

- Apply Melissa to the bottom of your feet or topically over your kidneys, liver, or throat. It can help remove emotional blocks, balance the emotions, and instill a positive outlook on life. Enjoy the unique lemony aroma.

Essential oils can be valuable, potent aids to promoting healing and wellness and can help remove energetic blockages of body, mind, spirit, and emotions. The oils are most effective when they are organic, thera-peutic-grade quality. Avoid heating these oils as heat destroys some of the beneficial properties.

Many of the oils can also be worn as a safe alternative to perfumes and colognes. They can be diluted with organic, food-based oils like almond oil. Some less expensive essential oils are only perfume-grade and have no therapeutic value.

The best way to learn which oils are right for your special health concern is either to buy a good reference book on the therapeutic use of essential oils or to consult with a complementary or alternative medicine (CAM) practitioner trained in the use of oils. Some oils, like lavender, can help with a wide variety of health concerns; others are for more specific uses.

More Steps to Tiger Freedom:

- Be willing to see yourself and the world differently. Ask for help in making this shift. Consider working with an energy medicine therapist, a spiritual counselor, a personal coach, or a psychotherapist.

- Push beyond your comfort zone. Stretch to the edge of your limiting beliefs and then stretch a little farther. Enjoy the freedom and the new feeling of empowerment that comes from releasing patterns no longer serving you.

- Try something new that may seem a little scary or weird. Share the experience with someone supportive of you.

- Give up the idea that someone has to be right and someone has to be wrong.

- Let go of "shoulds," feelings of rightness of your beliefs, behaviors, and opinions, and the wrongness of other positions that don't agree with yours.

Healing Guide

What are *you* doing to let go of fears and limiting beliefs? Choose something and focus on doing it on a regular basis. Remember that no one else and no thing outside yourself can control you.

As long as you come from your heart, that knowing, compassionate place deep inside, you are coming from a place of power. While others may not like what you share with them and may choose to act like a victim or even an aggressor, you can be at peace with yourself. And...you'll set your tiger free.

Tiger love is
unconditional
love.
To find love and joy,
look inside yourself
instead of searching
outside yourself.

CHAPTER TWO

Discovering the
Tiger's Love

Opening to Self-Love

HAVE YOU EVER LOVED SOMEONE who didn't acknowledge or reciprocate that love? At some time in your life, you may have felt a desire for love in a deeper, more fulfilling relationship. Perhaps you didn't fully understand what you were searching for.

Many of us seek approval, love, or fulfillment from other people, careers, activities, or material things outside ourselves. Some people live their entire lives never discovering where love is and why it seems to elude them. A popular country song includes the lyrics, "looking for love in all the wrong places." When I hear them I think, "How sad, but true."

Perhaps you have heard someone say, "If only I had _____, I'd be happy." You may even have said it yourself. Next time you hear yourself saying that or something similar, ask why you want that. When you get an answer, ask again, "Why do I want *that?*" Continue until you get to why you *really* want it.

To love and be loved is a deep universal need. If you ask a friend, a neighbor, or a family member what she really wants in life, she may say a new house, a new car, a good job, or even a meaningful relationship. If you take the time to probe deeper, you'll usually find that the underlying, unexpressed feeling is that she doesn't have the love she desires in her life. The second path on the journey is loving and respecting yourself and others.

Love is the essence of who we are. Think of it like a salmon's instinct to return to a special place to spawn. It seems compelled or guided to fulfill its journey, its life purpose. As humans, we also are guided to return to a special place of knowing within us. What if our life's purpose is to return to that place within of true peace, joy, and love?

Love is the **essence** *of who we are.*

Brenda's Story

When I think of empowerment, getting in touch with inner truth, I also think of some of my clients like Brenda. I have been seeing Brenda professionally on a regular basis to provide insight into her eczema and other health concerns. Eczema is a skin condition that manifests as red, rough patches in various places on the body, including the face.

Using a combination of muscle testing (applied kinesiology) and intuition, I determined that emotions played a significant role in Brenda's eczema. An energetic emotional release (EER) technique and Healing Touch helped clear the congested energy around the eczema.

One day Brenda came into my office and said, "I'm a mess! This eczema has spread out over most of my body." I asked what had been going on for her emotionally since I saw her last. She responded by saying her mother had been on her mind a lot lately.

Brenda continued, "I've been trying to figure out why my mother doesn't love me or show any affection toward me. Over the years I've come up with different ideas to try to explain that. I thought for years that I just needed to do more to please her. Then I thought she was jealous of me. My latest idea is that my mother is mentally ill."

"It's wonderful," Brenda continued. "I see now that it doesn't have anything to do with me. I have had this desire for love all my life. I have had the expectation that my family should provide that for me. Now I know that isn't true. It has nothing to do with the truth of who I am. Love comes from deep within me and not from anything outside of me."

Brenda's increased awareness of the body, mind, and spirit connection led her to this powerful insight.

One school of thought about eczema is that it may represent an intense desire for intimacy. In Brenda's case, the longing was for her parents' love and affection. When she changed her perception of where love is, she also realized that she was free of a past, restrictive emotional pattern. As long as Brenda bought into the old beliefs, she also felt something must be wrong with her. Now she no longer defines her self-worth by her perception of her parents' behaviors.

Once you get the message, as Brenda clearly did, you'll often find that physical symptoms either ameliorate or disappear completely.

Lots of people have difficulty finding and acknowledging the love deep inside themselves. Many clients have self-esteem issues. One of the things I suggest for changing that is saying the affirmation, "I love and accept myself just the way I am." That may sound very easy to you. If so, you'll be surprised at how challenging it can be for many people to make that simple statement and mean it.

Nearly all of my clients say, "But I *don't* love and accept myself." I tell them I believe that we are each created in the image of Spirit or a higher power. As such, our true nature is love. I suggest thinking of "myself" as "my Self" to focus on their God essence, their spiritual self. If this isn't comfortable for them, I offer a variation: "I am *willing* to love and accept myself."

After saying one of the above affirmations, or statements of belief, as though it's already happening, clients usually report noticing changes in how they view themselves. Some shifts are subtle. Some are more dramatic. The

"I love and accept myself just the way I am."

good news is that this often happens in a short period of time. An important part of effecting change is increasing awareness of your self-talk and of how you've been treating yourself.

When you discover some of the ways you've been diminishing your self-esteem, take some steps to let go of your old belief system, your old self-deprecating behaviors. For example, if you notice negative self-talk like: "You're such a loser," "You can't do anything right," or others from your personal examples, be easy on yourself. Notice what you just said. Then rephrase it in a positive way.

Saying something like, "I don't know why I always do that. I can never seem to get it right," reinforces the old pattern of self-abuse. Criticizing your actions or resisting them strengthens the behavior you're trying to change. When you catch yourself doing that, just allow it to be. It's already in the past. Make a loving statement about how you treat yourself, smile, and go on.

You may find some other examples helpful, such as: "I see what I just did. However, I choose to believe that _____." You can fill in the blank with whatever new behavior or image you really want to create. Consider making statements like, "I am capable and intelligent and use my power wisely." "I am agile and well-coordinated." "I speak easily and effectively in front of groups of people."

Lack of self-love is often paired with a lack of forgiveness. Forgiveness is letting go of judgments of yourself and others. Forgiveness is allowing and flowing with what is. Forgiveness is taking responsibility for your life experiences, your feelings, your thoughts, and your emotions.

Forgiveness
is allowing and flowing with what is.

Forgiveness is not offering a quick, insincere "Sorry!" It is not continuously dwelling on, remembering and holding onto the "bad" thing someone did. Forgiveness is not trying to gain control over someone through manipulation or playing games to get what you want. Forgiveness does not mean condoning or approving harmful behavior. It isn't allowing the situation or words to continue to affect you.

Energetically, lack of forgiveness contributes to dis-ease, illness, and suffering. An inability to forgive can eat away at our peace and sap our energy and power. We simply cannot be in a place of love and power and hold a grievance against someone.

We cannot love and hate at the same time. Hate and anger drain our energy and therefore, drain our power. So does unforgiveness.

Tiger Tale #1
The Golf Hazard

Assume for a moment that life is a game, a game of golf. There are many useful life lessons one can gain from golf, but possibly none so insidiously treacherous and destructive as the water hazard. Imagine yourself walking down the fairway, a fairway you have never seen before. You are searching for your metaphorical golf ball.

You encounter a water hazard. Peering into it, you find your ball in the water on the edge of a pond. You try to retrieve it, but it rolls down a steep incline into deeper water. This makes you a little angry, but you can still see it resting on the bottom. There's hope. As you reach to fish it out, your feet are starting to get a little wet.

Then, all of a sudden, something thrashes around, knocking your ball even deeper into the muck. You quickly determine that there is a huge alligator in there, and now you have some decisions to make. You can:

1. Decide that since your feet are already wet, you should wade into that pond and wrestle that alligator into submission because of the pain of your lost golf ball.

2. Resume play, continually blaming the alligator for your ruined golf game.

3. Back up, take the penalty stroke, drop a new ball, and enjoy the rest of the day.

It is surprising how many people choose #1. It would be funny if it weren't so sad. The truth is, the alligator never cared about your golf ball. He was just being an alligator. That is what he is. By blaming or trying to punish the alligator, all you accomplish is dragging yourself down into the muck with him. Choice #2 is equally non-productive. Why ruin a wonderful day, with so much beauty to be enjoyed, by mentally dwelling in the one place you really don't want to be in the first place?

Have you forgiven everyone and everything for what they did to ruin your life, according to your perception? Think about it for a moment. A typical list of possibilities includes an ex-spouse, partner, friend, parents, children, bosses, and many others.

The person you hold the grievance against is living life unaware of and unconcerned about your emotional attachment to past situations and interactions. When you are unforgiving, you only hurt yourself. You are the only one who is suffering. You are the only one responsible for your feelings and for healing the emotional pain going on inside you. You can't live in love and peace and attract what you want now if you're holding onto the old energy. Singing the old "she (he) done me wrong" song keeps you stuck in unforgiveness.

Now...what about you? Most of the time if you're finding difficulty forgiving someone, you're also having trouble forgiving yourself. You may loudly proclaim, "But I'm not the one who was wrong!" However, deep down you may feel or wonder if you may have contributed to the problem.

See which of these sounds familiar to you. "If only I hadn't said... Perhaps if I'd spent more time...Why did I ignore my gut feeling? Oh, my! What if I am part of the problem?" Rehashing the past serves no useful purpose and further drains your energy and strengthens the grievance. Wishing it hadn't happened isn't helpful either. You cannot change that.

Have you forgiven yourself for not being perfect in the eyes of the world? You may think you should be brighter, faster, taller, nicer looking, more personable, a better dancer, and have a smaller nose. However, none of that really matters. You are already a perfect spiritual being.

So how do you let go of unforgiveness? Start by being willing to totally face up to your role in what happened. Accept it without blame, and love and forgive that part. Change your perception of the situation or person. If you've been judging what happened as a bad thing or a terrible loss, look at it again. See the situation as an opportunity for healing yourself and for spiritual growth. Choose to see the gifts and blessings that have manifested since then.

Perhaps your values or priorities have changed so that you have less attachment to material things. Maybe if you hadn't lost your job, you wouldn't have gone back to school and gotten into a career field you love. You may not have met your loving, supportive partner if you had continued in your previous relationship. You may feel more grateful for the "little," seemingly insignificant, things in your life now.

You are already a perfect **spiritual** *being.*

Another way to let go is to decide to forgive. Simply declare your willingness to release unforgiveness. You don't have to know how. You don't need a plan. A little willingness sincerely expressed is a very significant step. Believe that it is already happening. Trust that your inner tiger has many ways to get your attention and facilitate change. It will help you find the path to love and peace.

Know that everything has already been forgiven: your darker thoughts, your actions, and your unforgiveness. It's only your thoughts and perceptions of how things and people should be, should look, and should respond that make you unhappy. They take you away from that place of peace and love within you. They also take you into negative beliefs about yourself and others. Remember…change your thoughts and you change the world around you.

If you can't see the sun, does it mean it's not there? Of course not! But if we let our thoughts gain control, it will be easy to get taken down into the feeling of being surrounded by ominous clouds or the dark night. The darkness makes it harder to see the bright colors and to believe the sun exists.

Just as with the temporary disappearance of the sun, you may not always feel the light and joy within yourself. We can see through the clouds and beyond the darkness into the inner light that is always shining within us. If you find that too challenging to do, just go back to expressing a willingness to change your thinking and release the lack of forgiveness and negativity. It will begin to shift, revealing peace and love, the true essence of who you are.

Now is the time to let go of whatever thoughts and emotions are dragging you down. Simply stop the blaming and faultfinding and start with forgiving yourself fully and completely.

When I first started working on my self-concept, I realized how tough I was on myself. Being a perfectionist-type person, I strived for perfection in everything and, of course, didn't measure up to my standards. One of my most frequent self-deprecating chastisements was "You're so stupid." I discovered that I wouldn't talk to my worst enemy (if I had one) the way I talked to myself. What a revelation!

How do others treat you? How do you feel you deserve to be treated? Let people know how you expect to be treated. Don't settle for less. A friend often says, "I am a princess." She doesn't live in a big castle or have a lot of money. However, she lives and behaves like a loving, empowered princess. She expects others to treat her like a princess, and they do.

Self-care is so important and is an integral part of self-love. Do you put everyone else's needs before your own, or do you nurture yourself by doing what makes you feel good about yourself? If you don't take care of your physical, mental, emotional, and spiritual needs, at some point you won't have enough of you left to give to others. If you're not making self-care a priority in your life, then you do not love yourself enough yet.

Janet's Story

One of the most memorable examples of self-nurturing I have seen occurred when I was taking a class onboard a ship on living life in a conscious, balanced rhythm. This class counted toward continuing education requirements. The instructor was Janet Mentgen, founder of the Healing Touch program.

Just before our lunch break, Janet told all of us in the class that she trusted we would all take care of ourselves in whatever way we felt guided to do. If we were drawn to engage in an excursion, an adventure, or a nap instead of returning for the afternoon portion of the class, she would consider that as an extension of the class. Basically, Janet was encouraging us to practice good self-care rather than just reading and talking about it. That is one lesson that everyone in the class remembered.

If you notice you haven't been doing anything to nurture yourself or to have fun, commit to doing at least one thing a week. Increase that to once a day, twice a day, and more. It doesn't have to take a lot of time or money, although you may want to splurge on yourself at least occasionally. You deserve it.

To feel **worthy** *and deserving, treat yourself as though you are.*

Consider dancing around your office or home for two minutes or singing a favorite tune or humming an original, spontaneous creation. Close your eyes, go to a peaceful, fun place in your imagination, and bask in that warm, peaceful feeling for a minute or more.

Go outdoors and walk briskly or leisurely around the building or parking lot at work or around the block, depending on time and weather.

It's amazing how quickly your energy level and thinking can shift with just a minute or two of focused self-nurturing. My point is that self-love manifests in many ways. It doesn't have to be expensive or time-consuming or take a lot of planning. Self-love is an attitude and a belief system that relates to self-worth. To feel worthy and deserving, treat yourself as though you are.

As you do more to focus on doing what feels good to you at a deeper level, you'll actually start feeling better about yourself. With a bit of intent, focus and practice, self-nurturing can be easy and frequent. Your self-love index will increase dramatically.

With your self-love meter turned on high, you'll feel more optimistic, energized, confident, courageous, and empowered. Now you can reach out to others with a higher energy vibration. You may choose to do some volunteer work by feeding the homeless, supporting women in need, or building or renovating homes for the poor. Do whatever you feel guided to do.

When we follow our passion and our joy, we'll have more than enough energy to work, play, and nurture ourselves and others. We'll attract more people who are positive, enthusiastic, and self-loving. We'll be more open to change and more willing to see situations and people, especially ourselves, in a new light.

Now...what about that meaningful relationship I alluded to earlier? Am I saying, "Forget the relationship? Who needs it?" Absolutely not! What I am suggesting is that we are more likely to attract a loving relationship with a significant other when we love and approve of ourselves.

You'll know you're coming from a place of power when you start appreciating the benefits of being alone. Sometimes this comes after several years of being alone.

You may have found a loving partner very early in life. If so, congratulations! You may truly like yourself and feel good about who you are. You may accept yourself without constantly judging what you do, criticizing yourself or playing the would-a, should-a, could-a game. You know the one. It's the one where no one ever wins and no one is truly happy, especially you.

Once you feel better about yourself, it's easier to access the love inside yourself and to share that with others. Now you're ready to consider entering into a meaningful relationship. When you know who you are at a deep level, and feel confident, courageous and empowered, you'll be clear about what you want and need in a relationship. You'll know where your boundaries are; which things you can compromise on and which you can't or won't. It will be easier to let go of any old beliefs about needing a man or a woman to be happy or to feel complete. You'll know you're already whole, complete, and loved.

You'll have the confidence to speak your truth, sharing from your heart without being so fearful about what effect that will have on your relationship. If he or she is not comfortable with that level of openness, then you may choose to take this as a sign that this isn't the one you're seeking. And, perhaps most important, you'll know if you need to walk away from a relationship, and you'll have the courage to do it.

You'll know you're already whole, complete, and loved.

If you continue to look outside yourself for love, you will always end up feeling disappointed, unhappy, and unfulfilled. Have you been searching for love in things or in relationships? Have you been holding someone else accountable for providing love in your life? When you finally realize that you don't need anything or anyone else to be happy, you are most likely to enter into a very loving, peaceful relationship. Tiger love is unconditional love.

Empowerment Guide

· You, and only you, are responsible for how much love and happiness you feel in your life.

- To feel loved, think love, breathe love, be love, give love, live love. Believe that love is the very essence of who you are.

- Forgiveness means letting go of judgments of ourselves and others, allowing and flowing with what is.

- Forgive yourself and others to feel more energized, lighter, more joyful and more empowered.

- To attract a loving, peaceful relationship, first love yourself and know who you are, what you need, and how to make choices from a place of power.

- Love yourself enough to take time to nurture your body, mind, and spirit.

- When we love and nurture ourselves consistently, we'll have enough energy left over to serve and help others.

Action Guide

Affirmations:

I connect with the source of love within which nurtures me in every moment.

I love and accept myself just the way I am.

I am the love I have been seeking.

Energy Technique:

Hold one hand over your heart. Focus your attention at your heart with your breath, feeling love energy expanding and warming you.

Stand in the grass in the sunshine. (I first heard this idea from a doctor.) Leather-soled shoes or no shoes work best. Close your eyes (or not) and feel the sun's rays beaming on you, coming through the top of your head, then filling your body and connecting with the earth through your feet. Continue to feel this energizing flow for one to three minutes or longer. Do it often. Getting a little fresh air and sunshine helps recharge your body, clarify your thinking, soothe your emotions, and recharge your spirit.

Inner Connecting: Tiger Love

Sit or lie quietly. Close your eyes and focus on your breath flowing freely and easily throughout your body. Visualize your breath and life force energy (chi) coming from deep in the ground up through your feet, through the core of your body. Continue through the crown of your head and beyond, reaching out to, and welcoming, that universal connection with Spirit.

Now reverse the flow, bringing your breath back down through the top of your head, the center of your body, your feet, and deep into the ground.

Bring your energy back up through the core of your body to your heart. Feel that energy as warm, loving energy growing stronger with each breath. Let that love energy expand to every part of your body, to every cell.

Feel love of the tiger within surrounding you. Let that feeling expand farther from your body, gradually encompassing everything and everyone in the world around you, everything seen and unseen. Bask in that warm, peaceful feeling of love for several moments.

Now, very slowly, bring your attention back to your breath. Feel love of self with each breath now and as you resume your daily activities. Start to feel your toes, then your fingers. Move them a little. Let your face form a smile, wiggle your nose, and open your eyes when you're ready.

As you become more familiar with this, you can shorten it to:

1. Close your eyes.
2. Be quiet and focus on your breath.
3. Feel love filling you, especially at your heart center, and expanding beyond.
4. Bring your attention to your breath.
5. Slowly open your eyes.

Ultimately, do whatever helps you get quiet and centered and feel loved and loving.

Essential Oils:

Rose, Ylang Ylang, Helichrysum or Angelica.

- Apply Rose or Ylang Ylang to the bottom of your feet and over your heart area to promote feelings of love and to attract love and joy.

- Apply Angelica or Helichrysum to the bottom of your feet and on your liver.

   You can also diffuse any of these into the air to help let go of angry, negative feelings.

More Steps to Tiger Love:

- Take time to pamper yourself by getting a gentle, relaxing Healing Touch treatment or a massage.

- Do something you enjoy, do nothing, or connect with the earth, your friends, your body, or your inner self.

- Exercise, eat healthy foods (organic if possible), take herbs and nutritional supplements, and drink plenty of filtered, purified, or spring water.

- Have fun, smile and laugh a lot. You'll look younger, more attractive, and more vibrant. Laughter also boosts your immune system and is very therapeutic.

- Get a pet (if you have time to properly care for it) or spend more time with the one you have. Pets love unconditionally and receive love in the same way.

- Look for shapes or figures in the clouds and watch them shape shift. Watch how the birds, squirrels, or ants move, work, or play.

- Dance (even if you don't know how), play an instrument, or just play or create something.
- Learn to do something you've always wanted to do.
- Look at your life with peaceful, loving eyes and give thanks for your life experiences (no matter how they appear to be).

Healing Guide

Have you truly forgiven yourself for your perceived shortcomings or the thoughts and actions you regret? To love deeply, you must first forgive. To forgive others, first forgive yourself. Since forgiveness and love are so closely interconnected, when you experience one, you'll experience both love and forgiveness.

If you are connecting with, loving, and trusting your inner self, you'll feel at peace with yourself and everyone around you. Forgiving and loving deeply and completely is empowering. People will feel your peace and strength and be attracted to you.

Speaking of
self-healing...
all of us are
healers.

CHAPTER THREE

Unleashing the
Tiger

Claiming Your Power

SO...BY THIS POINT ON YOUR JOURNEY, you know that the tiger within, your inner power, is always with you. You know you can tap into it and use it at any time. This third path is claiming your power.

Now let's look at some everyday situations that may drain your energy, perplex you, or worry you. We'll also focus on some ways to shift that by using your inner tiger.

Rachel's Story

RACHEL ASKED ME TO HELP HER with a "difficult situation." She explained that she was moving to another state soon and getting married. Rachel and her fiancé wanted to move into her rental house shortly after their arrival, but it was under a lease contract for another six weeks. Convinced that it wasn't possible to find anything to rent for that short period of time, Rachel was beginning to panic.

Rachel had asked the property manager to speak to the tenants and offer them an incentive for vacating the property early. Since he was unsuccessful, Rachel had decided to talk to the tenants personally but got knots in her stomach just thinking about it. Rachel had been giving her power to her tenants, blaming them for being uncooperative and causing her grief. She had felt the powerlessness and hopelessness of being a victim and of not listening to her "gut feelings." She was worried about how to get them to change their minds. "What can I say to them?"

"First," I replied, "it's possible that no words and no amount of money will get them to agree to move out early. Second, if you really want to talk to them anyway, then ask for guidance about what to say. Trust you'll know in the moment rather than trying to figure it all out ahead of time and worrying about it. It will help you let go of the knots in your stomach."

I continued, "You may want to look at the benefits of some of the other options. Since you're planning to do some remodeling in your house anyway, it might be easier and more pleasant for you to live somewhere else while the work is being done. You'll also be able to take your time moving in.

You can look at life as a gift— have fun with it.

Rachel had felt out of options, stuck and fearful. On the positive side, Rachel was aware of the signals from her body. She knew that what she planned to do didn't feel good to her. She did ask for help, an important step in empowerment. Rachel was open to, and considered, the guidance she had sought from me.

"You can look at this as a gift. Why not put some energy into what you really want, which is a nice place to live when you first arrive? Have fun with it!"

"Perhaps someone is going on an extended vacation and would like you to live in the house and take care of it. You can pursue other possibilities too; start asking people you know to make inquiries for you. You never know what will show up when you get clear about what you want and are open to new ideas."

Rachel responded enthusiastically with, "My sister has a friend who has had a house on the rental market for awhile. Maybe she'd be willing to rent to us on a short-term basis. I'll call her. I'm so grateful to you. The knots in my stomach are gone already!"

The change in Rachel in those few minutes was dramatic. Only her perception of the situation was different. She had been focused on needing a place to live since the tenants wouldn't move out early. Now she was open to other possibilities.

Now excitement and optimism emanated from Rachel's being and words. She exuded a sense of relief, peace, hope, and joy. Ultimately Rachel connected with, trusted, and used her inner power to guide her to the next step.

Francine's Story

Francine, a new client, asked for help in relieving the pain, allergies, and hives that covered her throat, shoulder area, and upper chest. In the first session I discovered, through intuition and an energy assessment, that much of the pain and allergic symptoms were related to emotional issues.

The energy at Francine's solar plexus, her energetic power center, was not flowing well. As I listened to Francine, I sensed a pattern of her feeling helpless in dealing with the men in her life. This "hopeless" situation started with her father. It continued with her husband and was reinforced by her current and former male bosses. All these men were, according to Francine, controlling, inconsiderate, and somewhat mentally and emotionally abusive.

Francine usually alternated between two coping responses. Either she said nothing, especially when it involved her father or her boss, or she lashed out verbally, often with her husband. This reactive behavior was not working for her. She was getting tenser and more depressed in spite of the medication she was taking and the psychotherapy she was pursuing. Her pain and hives continued to worsen.

When I suggested alternative, more empowering ways of responding to the men in her life, Francine was resistant and fearful. Over the next several months, we released some old emotional patterns. We also worked on improving her self-esteem. In addition, we talked about establishing healthy boundaries.

I asked Francine to consider her answers to questions like these...How do you feel when these men are being controlling and disrespectful? What contributes to that feeling? What can you do differently? What feels good to you and what doesn't?

> ## Know what nurtures and energizes you.

I suggested that Francine clearly define what she was willing to do and not willing to do. I continued, "Know how you desire and deserve to be treated. Know what nurtures and energizes you. How can you communicate this to these "controlling" men in a compassionate and yet powerful way? When you learn to do this, you can apply the same method to your coworkers, friends, associates, and children."

In a subsequent session, Francine decided to practice making more powerful statements with the men in her life. She chose to start by responding differently to her husband since he was the one she was the most comfortable with. She has been amazed and pleased with the results. Her husband has been treating her very respectfully, kindly, and considerately ever since.

When I last saw Francine, she had less pain than when I initially met her. The hives were better, but she still had some. She had not started making any power statements to any of the other significant men in her life.

Now let's look at how *you* can structure your time and your life differently. Prioritize your needs and activities. Let go of patterns and behaviors that don't feel good to you. Speak your inner truth.

Saying "No" is an extremely empowering response. Use it whenever you don't want to do something or don't feel good about it. Also use it if you are too busy to take on anything more. Resting or desiring more quiet time alone is very nurturing. Spending more time with family may be a higher priority than working late or meeting friends after work.

You do not have to justify your "No" or other choices. Another option you may offer is, "I've set priorities for my life. I'm focusing on what I need to do to take care of myself and my family." Otherwise, "No thank you," or "That's not going to work out for me now," is all you need to say.

Be very clear about your boundaries and what you need. Then decide if what those controlling people in your life are saying or asking fits into what is acceptable. If it doesn't feel good to you, it's time to speak up and share your truth with them. Setting boundaries and speaking your truth are very closely related and very important.

Perhaps you'll find some of the following responses helpful to you. "What you're saying (or asking) doesn't feel good to me. It feels like you're ordering me around (being disrespectful, putting me down, or taking advantage of me)." Use whatever fits your situation.

Then tell the person what you need. For example: "I need you to ask me respectfully to see if that works for me." " I need to be consulted (or considered) before you make a big financial decision that affects both of us."

Your power statements will vary according to the person or the specific situation. In some cases you may want to validate what was said. You can say, "Thank you for letting me know what you think. However, in the future I need you to bring it up with me as soon as you observe that instead of waiting until you're so upset. Then we can work on it together before it becomes such a big issue."

Now come up with your own statements based on your experiences and your boundaries. Know what will help you feel nurtured and peaceful. Adapt them to fit your personality so they sound genuine. Practice saying them. See which ones work for you. Discard or reword the ones that don't. It may help you to try them out on a friend or to say them aloud while looking into a mirror. You don't need to script your responses, but practicing some before you try this for real may give you more confidence. It can help you respond quicker and more powerfully when the situation arises.

If you're drawing people who are uncooperative or overly aggressive into your life, they may be reflecting something in you that you're not seeing or dealing with. It is even possible that you may be contributing to this kind of attack on a subconscious level. How you really feel about yourself, your job or your relationship may be expressing itself in a very subtle way.

There may be some issues you haven't wanted to address out of fear or because of your own low self-concept. Perhaps you choose to do something just to try to avoid conflict. By not speaking your truth, others may think you're uncommunicative, unable to deal with stress, or an easy target. Remember that others are our mirrors. They reflect something for us to look at and perhaps shift in ourselves.

Not speaking your truth can be less obvious also. On a very simple level, it can look like this. A friend or spouse asks you what you'd like to do this weekend. You had been planning to stay home to catch up on some things and relax. You say, "Oh, I don't know. What would you like to do?" When you are asked, "Where would you like to eat?" you say, "I don't care; anywhere is fine." The truth is you really want to go to the new restaurant across town.

Another form of not speaking your truth is even subtler. You don't like the way your spouse leaves her clothes all over the house, but you don't say anything. You start feeling resentful. You blame her for not being more considerate.

Here's another way you may be giving away your power. You really enjoy how your husband holds you closely and gently strokes your head and back. The problem you see is that he doesn't do it very often. Instead of telling him how much you enjoy it and asking him to do it more often, you feel unhappy and neglected.

These examples may sound familiar to you. "If he can't see that I could use some help, I'm certainly not going to ask for it." Then you become grumpy or uncommunicative. You feel stressed and pressed for time. He may be thinking that you must want to do the project by yourself since you didn't consult him about it or ask him for help.

Here's another one. "Can't she tell that I need some time to myself now? She keeps interrupting me when I just need to relax." You are stressed and irritated. You decide you're not getting what you need from this relationship. She's thinking that you don't love her any more because you're ignoring her.

If you aren't getting what you want, start asking for it. It's important to be able to talk about your needs calmly. Coming from a place of compassion without blaming the other person promotes healthy communication.

If you aren't getting what you want, start **asking** *for it.*

As a follow-up to the last scenario, you might say something like this. "Lately I've been feeling very stressed at work and irritated with my boss. I've finally figured out what I've been doing. I've been projecting that onto you. What I realize now is that I've been upset with myself for not letting you know what I need. After working all day in a stressful environment, when I come home I just need time to unwind by myself. So if you can give me about thirty minutes alone, I can be more present for you. Then we can share with each other. Will that work for you?"

Bobbi's Story

Speaking your truth also includes acting on what feels good to you in your day-to-day experiences. Recently I attended a conference comprised primarily of those in the healing professions. After sitting in a session with about five hundred people for part of one morning, I started feeling very tired and somewhat bored. The keynote speaker was reading a lot from her new book, and I needed to shift my energy.

I whispered to Bobbi, the woman next to me whom I had just met and been visiting with earlier: "Do you want me to get you anything? I'm going to get some coffee. Or would you like to come with me?" Bobbi asked me if it would be okay if we left. I assured her that it would be.

When we got outside into the hall, Bobbi said, "I feel so naughty leaving the session." I suggested that she might consider reframing that idea into something like, "I feel great when I do what feels good to me. I feel empowered by my choices." She agreed she would feel better thinking of it that way.

How do we give our power away? One way is by not using it to express our needs. When we allow others to control us or treat us disrespectfully or abusively, we are giving your power to another person or situation. We broadcast our feelings by our body language, such as with lack of eye contact, poor posture, and other signals. Such responses say that any unhappy people are welcome to "dump" on us.

We have the power to change that pattern. It's important to believe we can make a difference in how we're treated or in how our lives feel to us. When we feel good about ourselves, we are well on our way to using our inner power wisely.

Mary's Story

Now let's look at the situation Mary was facing. Mary lay down on my massage table one day and said, "I'm so confused. I don't know what to do. I hope you can help."

Mary explained that she and her estranged husband had been considering getting back together. "He wants to try it again. In some ways I'd like to also. However, I'm afraid he'll be unfaithful again. I won't tolerate that. I really need to get some clarity."

I assessed Mary's biofield energy system, checking the flow of life force or chi in and around her body. It felt strong and balanced. However, the energy around her feet and ankles was not flowing well. Emotionally this pattern indicates a lack of clarity in deciding what direction to go.

At the thymus or high heart, found above the heart, the energy felt very congested. It did not appear to be flowing freely through this area. As I placed my hand on the thymus, I sensed a partial blockage in the energy field. I intuited an emotional basis for this congested energy. In addition, I sensed that the initial cause went back to something that happened when

Mary was about nine years old. I knew it related to her friends at school and was not related to her classes. Whatever happened had felt overwhelming.

Mary suggested several possibilities, but none of them felt right. Then she said, "I know. Jumping! I could never jump. All the other kids could, but I never could figure it out no matter how hard I tried." That resonated with both of us.

From there we were able to connect the lack of ability to jump with feeling overwhelmed. Mary had tried to figure it out with her mind but only got more confused. She didn't know what to try, how to do it, or why she couldn't figure it out.

Since Mary couldn't resolve the dilemma or release the emotion around it as a child, feeling overwhelmed got "stuck" in her thymus. This is one of the places where that specific emotion typically gets stored. As other life experiences come along, the overwhelmed emotional response gets triggered more quickly. The energy in the thymus gets more congested and entrenched. Subsequently, the ability to consider other alternatives decreases.

When we release the emotional energy in an area of the body, it's easier to see the situation more objectively, with less emotion around it. It's easier to consider alternatives, get clarity, and connect with your inner guidance.

As I continued to hold my hand over Mary's thymus, I asked her to focus her attention deep inside her body beneath my hand while breathing in and out of that area. Feeling the emotion of being over-whelmed at nine and just allowing it to be—without resistance—helps break up the old pattern.

As the energy started shifting, I guided Mary to change her focus and allow the emotional energy to gently release from her body. When it felt like the energy had finished releasing, I asked Mary to visualize the opposite emotion. Next, I guided her to feel it filling the thymus, replacing the emotion of feeling overwhelmed.

For a follow-up activity, I suggested Mary quickly review her life, from age nine forward, as though she's watching it pass by while she's on a train. I asked her to look for those life experiences related to feeling overwhelmed. Increasing awareness of patterns, overwhelming experiences, and what creates fear is very helpful in initiating change.

She felt release, relief, and **peace.**

Mary and I talked about how confusing it can be sometimes to try to figure out the best option using only the left-brain. The left-brain likes to consider all the options that come to mind, research, think, and analyze. With lists of pros and cons and more and more data, and input from others, it can become very confusing. This is especially true for something with a strong emotional root.

Mary agreed to do other follow-up activities for gaining further clarity about what feels right in her relationship with her husband. The work we did together was a powerful step in helping Mary gain greater clarity and confidence.

Now here's the rest of the story. Less than a week later, Mary reported that she left my office with a great sense of calm. She felt release, relief, and peace.

Mary did some of the activities I suggested. Her awareness increased. She also talked to friends about her situation. She paid close attention to the words they used. One woman said, "Mary, you have your sparkle back." Another said, "You look great! You look like you've lost some weight."

Mary has a new realization. "It's only going to hurt me if I continue to be angry and upset about what he did. Now I know that I wasn't happy in my marriage. My husband has a lot of negativity that was affecting me. He needs to work through his stuff on his own. I can't help him with that."

Mary has been socializing, going to parties, and meeting new people. She said, "I'm having too much fun now. I don't know if we'll get back together. It really doesn't matter right now."

Perhaps you have wrestled with an overwhelming, worrisome, difficult, or fearful situation. You may have felt like you were all by yourself in a black hole with no way out. If you have, how did you deal with it? Disregarding your feelings and doing nothing is one option. You may have repeated the drama of the situation to everyone you met and asked others what you should do. Perhaps you worried and fretted in silence, letting your fears paralyze and depress you. Maybe you could see only one way of looking at it.

What did you do to resolve it? Perhaps you attributed it to "dumb luck" or circumstances beyond your control. Maybe you let someone else take over and "fix" it. Instead, you may have made yourself sick worrying about it.

If you or someone close to you is "playing" the role of the victim, some of these behaviors and coping mechanisms may sound very familiar to you. A victim usually stays in the same situation, allowing the same abusive person to play the role of aggressor or victimizer. If the victim leaves, she's likely to attract a similar situation or person because she hasn't looked at her role in creating it. She hasn't healed that aspect of herself. She hasn't set clear boundaries or used her power to help herself.

Culturally, there is a tendency to believe that men are the perpetrators and women and children are the victims. However, this is often not the case. In many situations men act as victims, feeling powerless to change anything.

The women in their lives may be physically, emotionally, or verbally aggressive; alcoholics; or control freaks. They expect the male in the relationship to do everything for them while giving nothing in return. Ladies, if you recognize yourself in any of these examples, take a close look at how you feel about yourself and your connection to Spirit. Men, if you are the abuser, look at what deep needs within you aren't being met. Counseling or therapy and energy work can be very helpful.

Now let's talk more about feeling you're the victim of a situation. First of all, you're never *really* the victim of circumstances although you certainly may feel like it at times.

One example of this is staying at a job you hate because you need the money. Another one is leaving a job, a home, and friends you enjoy to care for an ailing parent because you feel you "should." Finally, taking on too many activities is draining your energy and your joy. However, you feel compelled to continue with them because you made a commitment. You don't want to let anyone down. Situations like these may leave you feeling helpless and hopeless.

If you are acting like a victim, feeling powerless, know you always have choices. You can stay in the same situation or relationship and do nothing. However, this option will continue to drain your energy physically, emotionally, mentally, and spiritually. It will give you more of what you don't want. An old saying comes to mind that is relevant here: *If you continue doing what you've always done, you'll continue to get what you've always gotten.*

Another choice is to stay in the situation and see it differently (unless it involves physical abuse.) You can seek help from a counselor, personal coach, support group, or an ongoing spiritual gathering; or spiritual books, videos, and DVDs. Also, you can draw on your inner power and faith to ask for guidance and a new way of seeing the "problem" or situation.

A third option is to leave the situation or relationship. It may be helpful to give yourself some time and space away from your concerns to get more clarity and become more peaceful. Take time to get in touch with how you really feel and what you desire. Discover what you need to feel nurtured and heal those old wounds.

Focusing on self-healing is the single most useful thing you can do to bring more peace and joy into your life. Find out what you think you really deserve. When you are valuing yourself, speaking your truth, and respecting others, you energetically send out a message of self-assurance and self-worth. That's what you'll be attracting. We'll talk about this in more detail in Chapter Six.

Speaking of self-healing...all of us are healers. Some of us facilitate healing professionally and some as an avocation. However, healing is an inside job. We all do it. It's one of our innate gifts and abilities. When we hold a painful part of our body, we feel better. We do it instinctively whether we have any special training or not.

Healing is different from curing. Physicians focus on curing an illness or alleviating a symptom. A doctor can set our broken leg, but our body repairs the injury. True healing and power come from deep within, through our inner tiger. That guidance shows us how to see the world with the eyes of peace and truth.

Troy's Story

Troy, who's a surgeon, came to me because of severe pain in his feet that he'd had for ten years. He didn't want the surgery the other doctors had recommended. After one session, Troy's pain was nearly gone. By the third session, he had resumed normal activities and was nearly pain-free.

Stuart's Story

Stuart is an elderly gentleman who came to me complaining of severe pain around his heart and chest. The doctors told him he'd either need to live with the pain or have expensive surgery. I used a variety of energy techniques to help shift the energy and release the pain related to his heart, chest, and back. I also used some crystals to help release the congested energy. By the end of the first session, the pain had greatly reduced. Stuart was very interested in learning more about the healing properties of crystals

> *True* **healing** *and power come from deep within, through our inner tiger.*

and stones and how energy healing works. I suggested some resources for him to explore. I also showed Stuart how to hold his hand over his heart and chest to help release the pain.

At the beginning of the second session, Stuart reported that he had been using the technique with great success. He said he also discovered that he could use that same procedure to relieve pain anywhere in his body. He was getting the same good results whenever he placed his hands somewhere with the intent to release the pain. He was excited about this and motivated to learn more ways to help himself and others. He was also drawn to purchase some crystals and was using them to help balance his energy.

Stuart is truly claiming his power, facilitating his own healing and learning what alternatives to traditional health care are available. Because Stuart has so much less pain now, he's resuming a more active life and planning to see me again when he feels a need for my help and isn't quite so busy.

Health care is a critical place to speak your truth. Your choices directly affect you and your family. My heart goes out to people who don't believe they have any options in health care. They are often so locked into their old patterns, beliefs, and fears that they won't seek any alternatives to traditional, allopathic medicine.

I used to think mainstream medicine was the only way to go. That was before I became critically ill. Then as I became sicker and sicker, I realized that even the specialists didn't have a clue how to help me. That's when my search for answers led me to explore and benefit from the wonderful world of complementary health.

Now I see clients who are claiming their power and seeking alternatives to surgery and drugs. They are seeking help and support for self-care and wellness. If they want a diagnosis, drugs, surgery, or high-tech, they know traditional medicine is the place to go. Forming partnerships with your health care providers is an empowering way of approaching health care.

How do you choose your physicians and complementary health care providers? How do you know if they're right for you? What can you do other than blindly follow whatever they tell you to do? I address these and other questions and share more client stories and details about my health care journey in another writing entitled *Tiger Health: Choosing Wisely.*

Now is the time for you to take charge of your life, take responsibility for your choices, and create what you want. You may be saying, "It sounds good. I'm ready, but what do I do next?"

Now is the time to reveal the great secret you've been keeping. It's a secret you've kept so well for so long you may not even remember it. Let me refresh your memory. The great secret is...you really do have a tiger within.

Go deep inside yourself and look around. You'll surely find the tiger. Everyone has one. See what your tiger is doing. Perhaps it's awake and playing. On the other hand, your tiger may seem only half awake or may be partially hidden from view. If you've been ignoring the tiger or pretending it's asleep, now is the time to realize the tiger is fully awake.

The great secret is...you really do have a tiger within.

And there's more good news. If you don't feel ready or motivated to change your life, that's up to you. You can continue as you are for now, perhaps half-asleep to the truth of who you are. You get to choose.

If you sense there has to be more to life than what you've been experiencing, you've already made a good start. If you're looking for your life's purpose, you are acknowledging a power or energy beyond your body that guides you. This inner tiger gives you courage and moves you along on this metaphorical journey.

See your tiger as fully awakened now. Say, "I've been dreaming. Now I know there's another way of looking at these life experiences. There's another way of being, another source of courage and light." Accessing the tiger within is empowering. When you connect with the tiger within, you'll also be connecting with the courage to speak your truth, make empowered choices, be still and listen, and follow your guidance.

When we're asleep, we don't see the light. The same is true metaphorically. When we awaken to the tiger, we will be able to see the light. The light guides us and allows us to take bigger steps with confidence and knowing. We have a much better sense of where we're going. It's amazing how much easier life can be when the path is well lit.

Joy's Dream

One of my dreams relates to this feeling of confidence and self-assuredness.

> *I am walking by a church when a priest I know and like comes outside and walks over to me. Instead of his usual clerical garb, the priest is wearing a very bright, bold, patterned jacket and pants in turquoise and orange with a little black and white. I've never seen him in anything so bold before. He says, "I decided it was time to do something different and have a little fun."*

To me this dream, entitled "Priest Inspires Others to Make a Bold Power Statement," symbolizes empowerment. The priest represents the spiritual aspect of ourselves. The priest no longer feels compelled to follow his practice of dressing or acting in the way he has always done. The bold colors and patterns he now chooses to show to the outer world make a powerful statement of who he is inside.

Are you ready to gather up the courage to make your bold statement reflecting who you really are? Think of the fun you can have acting out and speaking your truth. You'll very likely be saying, "This is the new me, and I'm happy with myself."

"This is the new me, and I'm **happy** *with myself."*

Begin working with some of the Guides at the end of this chapter. In the next chapter and those following, you'll find more ideas and encouragement for awakening and seeing differently. You'll discover what feels best to you. Other ways of connecting with your inner power will surface as you

Essential Oils:

Fir and Ylang Ylang.

- Fir enhances the feeling of strength and power. Apply it to the bottom of your feet and to your solar plexus area. You can also diffuse it into the air.

- Ylang Ylang promotes a feeling of confidence, joy, and peace. Apply it the same as for Fir above.

More Steps to Tiger Power:

- To see someone differently, change your mind. Focus on seeing how others are like you, seeing their true essence or the light inside them. Try imagining them as a vulnerable child or someone's gentle, beloved grandmother.

- Look at difficult situations as growth opportunities. If that seems too difficult, practice the energy technique above.

- Do what you can for yourself. Then ask for help from others when you need it.

- If your mind is confusing, overwhelming, and stressing you, slow down and do some inner connecting.

- Distinguish your "stuff" from their "stuff." Avoid taking on what's not yours even though others may try to suck you into solving their problems.

- Pay close attention to what others are saying to you. They may provide clues to what's going on with you, how they see you, and what you may want to change.

- Make a bold power statement that reflects who you are or what you need.

Healing Guide

How do you currently see your world? You can choose to feel victimized and helpless or you can empower yourself. You can use your "old" physical eyes and continue to see the past and judge the present and the future accordingly. Or you can choose to see peace with your spiritual eyes. Change starts with heightening your awareness, desiring a change, and being willing to believe it's possible. It's up to you.

Paying attention to signs,
synchronicities, roadblocks,
detours, and unusual
occurrences is a good way
to start "tuning in"
to your
guidance.

CHAPTER FOUR

Letting Your
Tiger Lead

Following Your Inner Guidance

EVERYONE IS INTUITIVE—EVEN YOU.

Now let's take a closer look at using your inner tiger to connect with and follow your guidance. Following your inner guidance is the fourth path. This may come as a surprise to you, but *you* are intuitive. How do I know this? It's not because I'm so intuitive. Everyone is intuitive. You were born with that ability. However, you may not be aware of it, and you may not actively "tune into" it.

You may be saying, "But I'm not intuitive," or "I used to be intuitive when I was little, but I'm not any more. You may be wondering, "How am I supposed to connect with my guidance? It doesn't seem to work for me."

Another way to think of guidance is as an etheric, unseen bridge between us and Spirit, or a higher power, to help build that connection. That bridge is always in place. The bridge leads to peace and inner power. We can cross the bridge as often as we desire. Mayans and Native Americans, the red race, refer to the rainbow bridge as the connection between the Great Spirit and all relations and between the ancient ways and the modern world.

Your awareness of the bridge is different from anyone else's. It may vary anywhere along a continuum from no bridge to a weak bridge to a well-used one. Your sense of the bridge may change over time. You may notice a pattern of evolving into more familiarity with the bridge, more trust in it, and greater use of the bridge.

You may start seeing more colors in the bridge. You may feel more love energy as you're crossing it. One day you may cross the bridge to peace and choose to stay in that place of continuous connection with Spirit, that place of inner power.

The Four "Clairs"–Intuition

Next let's talk about what I call "the four clairs": clairaudience, clairvoyance, clairsentience, and claircognizance. Most commonly, these power tools are referred to as intuition. Intuition is an effective way of connecting to your guidance.

Here's an in-depth look at each of these "clairs" in everyday terms. The "clair" in each means clear.

Clairaudient:
Words or Sounds

You may hear sounds, music, or words that no one else hears. You may hear a long message or a single word or phrase. You may describe it or think of it as "a voice in my head." And no, you're not crazy. It's a perfectly natural ability.

You may be looking for clarity in some aspect of your life situation when you hear the lyrics of a song that answers your question. You may start singing a song repeatedly until you really listen to the words and relate it to your concern. An acquaintance may say something that gives you an idea. You may overhear a piece of a conversation that inspires or helps you.

If you are clairaudient, chances are you are very sensitive to noise and sound. You may need the volume on the radio or television lower than others do. You may feel most comfortable with soft, quiet music or no sound.

I sometimes get audient messages when I am working with clients. I share these with my clients with their permission.

Joan's Story

One day as I was holding Joan's feet while she was lying on the massage table, I kept hearing "violence." I was reluctant to share this with her since she was a new client, but the energy at her feet would not release. I finally asked permission to share with her. "I keep hearing the word 'violence,'" I said. She replied, "That makes perfect sense." The energy at her feet released, and we continued the session.

This message was for her and not me. I didn't need to know the details. However, my sense was that as a child she witnessed violence.

Sleep Related Audient Messages

Another time I receive audient messages is at night after I've been sleeping. I wake up briefly, hear the message, and go back to sleep. I always remember the message in the morning. And...I always pay attention to the message and follow through with what I'm to do.

One night I awoke suddenly, fully alert, and heard, *"You are going to the Yucatan."* It was a very loud, clear voice. This message seemed rather strange to me since I had no previous desire to go to the Yucatan. However, I started paying attention to the other signs and messages from people, including information on a women's spiritual retreat to the Yucatan in ten weeks. Funds for the trip became easily available. Everything fell into place effortlessly.

Very recently, after asking for guidance about the title for this book, I received another sleep related voice message *"Awaken the tiger!"* which I have used metaphorically throughout this book and as part of the title.

Clairvoyance:
Seeing

You clearly see an image, a symbol, or an event in your mind. You may have a sense of what they mean, which you then can translate into words. These could come in the form of a dream, a vision, or a waking moment. They may seem so clear you'll think it actually happened in form. Some clairvoyants "see" an event just before it happens, years before or as it occurs.

As a clairvoyant you may see small sparkling lights or flashing lights. These sometimes indicate the presence of angels or guides. You may see auras or energy fields around someone else's body, or your own, or around objects. You may see colors in the aura or see a bright white or yellow light.

If your primary "clair" is through vision, you'll very likely be more sensitive to light, colors, beauty in nature, or other visual compositions. You can visualize easily. Pay attention to what you see that catches your attention.

Clairsentience:
Physical Or Emotional Feeling

Clairsentients feel on many levels. You get "gut feelings." You know when something you are considering feels wonderful and peaceful or lousy and fearful. You may get a tingling feeling that I refer to as "Spirit tingles." You know the ones. They're a little like the goose bumps you get when you're cold only there's a sense of hearing truth or recognizing something profound. Sometimes you'll have a strong feeling that something feels right or wrong for you, but you can't explain it.

As a clairsentient you may feel a subtle pressure or have an awareness that something unseen is present. It may be an angel, a guide, or some other energy form.

"Feeling" people connect easily with people and places by sensing what the energy feels like. However, you probably don't think of it in those terms. You may say things like "I don't feel good in this place. I get a bad feeling here. I need to get out of here." Or you may say, "I feel really good when I walk in the park."

In a shopping mall or large public gathering, you may say, "There are too many people here for me. There's too much going on." You may feel that your energy is being drained. It can be challenging for you to keep from feeling too much of other people's energy. Chances are you'll usually try to avoid crowded places.

You enjoy being touched. Touching people, animals, and things feels good to you. You may be drawn to put your hands on someone to help them feel better. You could be attracted to the healing arts, fine arts, or other fields that involve extensive use of your hands.

Claircognizance:
Knowing

You know things that you can't explain based on facts or reasoning. You know beyond your years, learning, and experience. You say, "I just know," when asked to explain, or "It just came to me." Your messages may take the form of instant knowing, an inspirational flash, a creative twist, a sudden solution to a problem, or a wonderful idea. You may be very intellectual and analytical and drawn to fields like science, mathematics, and computers.

Some people have a primary "clair" with lesser-developed abilities in others. Can you identify with one or more of these forms of intuition? Your ability may not feel strong at first. However, with practice and focus you can improve it much like you build weaker muscles when you exercise them regularly. Please refer to the Action Points at the end of this chapter for activities for building your intuition.

If you don't recognize yourself in any of these forms of intuition, it's okay. Not everyone has developed the ability to connect with divine guidance in this way. You may relate easier to some of the other forms of guidance we'll be talking about next.

More Power Tools

Now I want share some additional "power tools" with you. I find these useful in strengthening the connection with the rainbow bridge described at the beginning of this chapter.

Prayer:

One of the most commonly accepted and used techniques is prayer. Prayer takes many forms, from rote recitation of religiously proscribed prayer to a simple feeling, a statement of trust or intent to help others. Sometimes we may feel our prayers have been answered and sometimes, because we didn't get what we asked for or weren't listening carefully, we may feel our prayers weren't answered.

Some feel prayer is a communion with Spirit or All That Is. The name for that presence or power that guides you varies from one culture, one religion, and one individual to another. Substitute whatever name you are most comfortable with.

Dreams:

Dreams can be wonderful tools for receiving guidance. Pay attention to your dreams. Learn what the symbols in dreams may mean. However, while many books on the meaning of dreams are available, keep in mind that dream interpretation is specific to the dreamer: you. You may find taking a class on dream work or joining a local dream group helpful.

Paula's Dream

One day I was working with Paula on using and following her guidance. It was then that she shared this recurring dream with me.

> *I am at an art gallery. An artist has made a very large abacus. I, along with several others, am trying to agree on the best way to display it. Some suggest it be done symmetrically; others say it should be placed on end; still others want it on an angle.*
>
> *Finally, one of the men gets inside the abacus and changes the way it's arranged. He gets out and everyone is satisfied. He could control it from the inside but not from the outside.*

Paula was puzzled by her dream and didn't get much from it. When I searched for a message in this dream, I sensed that when I look at something from the outer, worldly perspective, I may see and feel dissension, confusion, and tension. It's only when I remember to go inside and be quiet that I find easier resolution, clarity, and peace.

You may get a different message, and that's okay. Whatever you get from your dreams is right for you in that moment.

You can learn many techniques for getting guidance from your dreams. A very simple one is to set your intent, just before you go to sleep, to receive guidance on a specific area of concern. When you do that, you'll often get insight, clarification, or inspiration that is helpful. If you don't recall the dream, ask again—and ask to remember and understand the dream message.

Messages:

Calling on angels, saints, or spirit guides to provide messages, insights, or help with specific issues or concerns can be very helpful. For example, Archangel Michael is considered to be the angel of protection while Archangel Raphael is the angel of healing. These special beings may intercede and answer our prayers, send us a sign to let us know they are nearby, or give us a message or a nudge so we'll know what to do.

Inner Connecting:

Meditation is a very powerful tool for connecting with your guidance. Think of it as "inner connecting." Let go of any idea you may have about how it "should" look. Get rid of the fear of doing it the "right" way.

If you have the belief that meditation is one of those "New-Agey" ideas or is too "woo-woo," set that aside also. Meditation or inner connecting is an ancient practice. The Bible refers to it as, "Be still and know." It can be used as a peaceful way to start your day or as a calming retreat from the busyness and concerns of your day.

"Be still and know."

Many books have been written about how to meditate; how often and where. Guided meditation tapes and CDs for facilitating inner connecting are abundant. Quiet music, nature sounds, or chanting help some people relax and quiet their minds. Sitting in silence in a peaceful place in your home, in a church, or outdoors on a special rock or propped against a tree may help you with inner connecting.

As a child living with my elderly grandparents, I used to go out often in the wooded area of their farmland and climb high in a tree. I thought about nature, God, or nothing at all. Sometimes I asked myself questions for which there were no answers. I certainly didn't call that meditation at the age of six or nine years. Yet that's exactly what I was doing. My grandmother had to cut the pitch out of my hair so often she *almost* stopped scolding me about it.

You may prefer meditating in the bathtub surrounded by candlelight and bubbles, as one of my male clients does, more than sitting in pitch-laden trees. Some people like to burn incense or use essential oils as an aid for getting into a quiet space. A friend meditates in his car at lunchtime.

Walking in a quiet area such as the mountains, by the seashore, or other natural environment works well for some, especially those who have difficulty sitting still. Journeying is a form of inner connecting with focused intent used in the Native American tradition. Usually a soothing beat of the drum accompanies the process of connecting with animal guides and other guides.

You can do inner listening with a partner or group, or alone. You can set an intent for your inner connecting or just still your mind and be with whatever shows up for you. When thoughts appear, watch them without resistance and gradually come back to stillness. You can meditate daily or less often. It's up to you. Regular meditation helps you be more peaceful and centered. You may be able to put things into perspective more easily.

When thoughts appear, watch them without resistance and gradually come back to **stillness.**

While you may find some of these inner-connecting methods helpful, you will not automatically be able to do inner connecting by using any of these physical aids. However, you may want to experience some of these techniques. See which one(s) resonate with you.

The bottom line is that meditation is a very individual thing. It is a practice or method of going into the stillness, letting go of the confusion, stress, and beliefs that keep your spirit hostage. With more practice you may find you can go to that quiet place inside you with greater ease. You'll discover how meditating is helping you.

Through inner connecting, we can find peace and clarity. Meditation is just one power tool for facilitating our sense of connection with our inner tiger. Ultimately life is to be lived in a continuous state of inner connecting. Stillness, peace, love, and inner knowing are our natural state.

Observation:

Another "power tool" is to observe keenly. Listen to the spaces between the words. Listen to what isn't being said. If you start thinking of your response and questions while someone is talking, you'll miss a lot of subtleties.

Practice seeing beyond the physical body and your surroundings. See deeper into the spirit of the individual. Pay careful attention to body language. Does this person make eye contact? Do you feel a sense of ease or dis-ease about the person? Do you get a "good" feeling about being with this person or being in this place? What is your first impression? It's often right on target.

Practice **seeing** *beyond the physical body and your surroundings.*

Women have a definite advantage over most men in "reading" people and situations and gathering information through observation, subtle clues, and intuition. Have you ever had this conversation or a similar one with someone?

She: Did you notice how nervous Joe was tonight? Something's wrong.

He: No. What makes you think so?

She: Didn't you see how he kept looking around as if he expected someone to sneak up on him? And did you notice how he kept fidgeting in this chair and looking at his watch?

He: No.

She: And he was perspiring a lot even though the room was cool.

He: I guess I didn't notice that either, but none of that means anything.

You, as the woman, are forming impressions that have nothing to do with what Joe said. You, as a man, are more focused on what was being said and the grosser aspects of that encounter. I commend the men who also observe closely and use the subtler forms of communication effectively.

Paying attention to signs, synchronicities, roadblocks, detours, and unusual occurrences is one of the easiest ways of "tuning in" or receiving guidance. I'm quite certain most of you know what I'm talking about.

Real-life examples are plentiful. You've felt drawn to take a trip to visit your ancestral homeland and help a chronically ill elderly relative. However, you haven't made any plans yet because you work full-time and don't have the extra funds to make the trip.

One day you receive a large settlement check in the mail for an insurance claim you made long ago. Since you now have extra funds, you decide to see if you can get time off from work. Surprise! Your company has been considering doing some temporary layoffs and your request is gladly approved. I believe you were being guided and helped to do what you sensed was right but weren't doing due to fear or doubt.

Work with the roadblocks that may come up occasionally. Look for the messages they can give you. Here's an example.

Joy's Story
Detours and Delays

I was working on a program of study to become certified as an instructor. Most of the requirements revolved around observing other instructors, co-teaching, and finally, teaching a class under supervision.

Shortly after I began, I started experiencing one detour, delay, or roadblock after another. Classes were cancelled or rescheduled at a time that didn't work for me. One classroom facility was being remodeled. Another time I arrived at a college out of town only to find the class had been cancelled due to illness in the instructor's family. One of my personal favorites was when a college that regularly offered the class forgot to list it in the course catalog—for the first time ever!

Some of you, by now, may have given up on this goal or gotten the inner message that this wasn't working out very well. Not me! I continued following the detours and promoted and planned for the big event—solo teaching. Four people pre-registered. Five was the minimum for holding the class.

I asked the supervising instructor the procedure for getting reimbursed for the promotional expenses for the class. She said, "I don't know. It's never happened to me before." Now *that* got my attention.

Finally, I found out that the anatomy and physiology classes that I had taken previously didn't meet the requirement for this program. Until I took a college class in anatomy and physiology, I would not be eligible to be approved as an instructor.

That's when I really knew, without a doubt, and accepted that it wasn't meant to be. In spite of the time, money, and effort expended, it was time to let it go.

Have you ever met up with roadblocks that finally convinced you that you were being guided to take a different path? Your experience may have revolved around a relationship, a job, or trying to buy a house you thought was perfect for you. Perhaps what appeared to be roadblocks were really detours or messages telling you to try it a different way. Your tiger guide may have been saying, "Whew! I had a tough time getting through to her, but she finally got it."

Signs:

Another "power tool" is noticing the signs in your life. A sign can be as simple as hearing the name of a health practitioner who is very successful in helping people relieve allergies. You hear the same name with favorable comments twice more in as many days. Since your son has severe allergies, you decide you'll call her and make an appointment.

You see a sign that says "Slow Down" when you've just gotten news of a heart problem or a job layoff. You feel guided to take time off, go on a vacation, and start writing the book you've been intending to write.

Have you ever thought about calling someone when the phone rings, and it's the person you were thinking of? Have you wanted to talk to a friend and haven't found the time to call? Then when you stop at a gas station on the other side of town, there she is getting gas. It turns out that she's free for lunch and so are you.

The above examples fall under synchronicity rather than coincidence. Coincidence suggests a chance occurrence. These friends were both guided to be in the same place at the same time. The guidance was subtle but very effective.

You may have heard stories similar to this next one.

Tiger Tale #2
Plane Synchronicity

You need to catch a plane this morning. You drop a bottle of juice on the floor and stop to clean up the mess. As you're closing your suitcase, you realize your underwear is still in the dryer. At the last minute, you can't find your keys. Ten minutes later they show up in their usual place. An accident on the freeway slows you down another fifteen minutes.

You guessed it. You miss your plane. If you're in your power, you can flow with the delay and calmly reschedule. If not, you may be stressed, worried, or angry. In either case, when you learn that the plane you were to have taken has crashed, you are grateful. Your guides, guidance, or intuition was at work, slowing you down enough to keep you from being on that plane.

The above example relates to detours and signs as well as unusual circumstances. They are also examples of recognizing guidance and flowing with it even when you haven't specifically asked for any help.

Being aware of and open to guidance is very helpful. It's even more helpful to listen to and follow your guidance. Here's another story to illustrate this point.

Tiger Tale #3
Willie's Story

A great flood was destroying property and causing people to relocate to safer areas. Law enforcement officials and teams of volunteers were contacting people to tell them they needed to leave the area. The water was rising rapidly. People were leaving quickly by any transport available.

Willie, whose house was being flooded, prayed to God to save him. A canoe came by and a man asked Willie if he wanted to come with him. "No, God will save me."

An hour later, as the water was rising higher and higher, a boat came by, and a volunteer called to Willie to come aboard. "No thank you. God will save me."

Willie finally was forced to climb onto the roof of his house to avoid the water. A helicopter hovered overhead, and a man yelled out, "Grab hold of the ladder, and we'll take you to safety."

"No thank you," says Willie. "God is sending me help."

Moments later as Willie arrives at the pearly gates, he calls out, "God, I thought you were going to save me!"

A big booming voice calls back, "Who do you think sent you the canoe, the boat, and the helicopter?"

Are you like Willie at times, dismissing the help, comforting words, and support of other people?

Spirit, the All That Is, uses other people, events, signs, synchronicities, and symbols to get our attention and guide us through life. It's time to start tuning in to how your guidance is manifesting.

Empowerment Guide

- Guidance comes in many forms. Intuition is one type of guidance.
- We can connect with our guidance and intuition in a variety of ways.
- We can strengthen our intuition by practicing, much the same as we become stronger when we work out.
- Four major forms of intuition are clairaudience, clairsentience, clairvoyance, and claircognizance.
- Use the four "clairs" and your power tools often: listening, seeing, knowing, feeling, prayer, dreaming, journaling, observing body language, following hunches, inner-connecting, setting intent, synchronicity, and noticing signs.

Action Guide

Affirmation:

I listen to and follow my guidance easily and frequently.

Energy Technique:

Sit or lie in a quiet place with your spine straight. Close your eyes and lightly touch your third eye, located just above the bridge of the nose. Focus your attention on this spot for a minute or two or more. When you do this daily, you may notice your inner awareness and intuition increasing. You may feel calmer and more at peace with yourself and the world around you.

Inner Connecting: Tiger Guidance

Sit quietly to do inner listening with the tiger within. Ask for your special guide or angel to come closer and help you with clarity. Ask a question or set your intent and wait. You may or may not get an answer immediately. Watch for forms of guidance such as signs, changes, or messages from others. Thank the tiger for the guidance as though you've already received it. When you are ready, bring your attention back to your breath, your physical body, your hands and feet, and the space around you. Open your eyes and smile.

Essential Oils:

Frankincense and Cedarwood

- Apply Frankincense to the bottom of your feet or diffuse into the air to open and enhance spiritual communication.

- Apply Cedarwood to the solar plexus, top of the head, back of the neck, behind the ears, or the wrist areas. Using Cedarwood can enhance the potential for spiritual communication and feelings of strength and empowerment. You may also diffuse it into the air.

More Steps to Tiger Guidance:

- Start paying closer attention to how you pick up hints, cues, and subtle information. Then work with developing that intuitive strength further.

- Pretend you can see more than you see with your physical eyes, hear what others don't hear, feel beyond your physical sense of touch, and know what your mind doesn't know. Then practice by checking the accuracy of what you've imagined.

- Take three playing cards, noting what they are, and mix them up. Place them face-down, side by side, and choose the one you've specified, e.g. the ten of hearts. When you select the correct one more often than chance, increase the number of cards you're working with and repeat. Practice with someone else telling you what card to find. Try it with one colored dot or symbol on small pieces of paper. Then find a specified color. Make up your own versions.

- Journal your thoughts, feelings, passions, and inspirations. Do this without analyzing, criticizing, editing, or judging. No one will be grading your spelling or grammar or even reading it. I recommend this as a daily practice. Go back and reread days, weeks, or months later to see if anything resonates with you differently than when you first wrote it. Does it inspire you or give you new direction or insight into how you really feel?

- Begin journaling your dreams. Set an intent to get clarification or insight into a situation, problem, or decision you've been trying to make. Use a book on dream symbolism or do a word association about the symbols in your dreams. Here's an example. An association for "kite" could be: fly, high, trees, sky, wind, childhood, fun, free. There's no right or wrong. Use the ones that ring true for you and fit best with the dream. Pay careful attention to the emotions in the dream. Look at who the people in your dream represent in your life. What are they doing? How are they acting? What can you learn from that?

- Observe a person's body language. Use the clues you pick up to supplement what you are hearing and sensing beyond the physical realm.

Healing Guide

We receive guidance all the time. If you aren't aware of it, focus on receiving your guidance more clearly. As you practice working with your guidance more and more, you'll be able to use it to help you make many day-to-day choices. Using it in this way will bring you greater confidence and peace.

Harmony

*and balance
are important in
every aspect
of our lives.*

CHAPTER FIVE

Connecting with the
Total Tiger

Harmonizing Mind, Body, Spirit

HARMONY AND BALANCE are important in every aspect of our lives.

Allopathic doctors are becoming more and more aware of the effect of the mind and spirit on the physical body. Stories abound about people recovering from illnesses when doctors have exhausted their resources and given up hope. The doctors usually say something like "It's a miracle," or "We can't explain how that happened."

What made the difference for the person who survived a death sentence? Sometimes it seems that it's prayers or other spiritual influences. Other times it may be related to sheer determination or intent. It can also be related to emotions. "I have two small children, and I really felt I couldn't leave them yet," provides a strong purpose for living.

Most complementary health practitioners actively focus on balancing and connecting body, mind, and spirit in our work with clients. Both practitioners and clients believe in the value of using a holistic approach to healing. The fifth path is balancing body, mind, spirit, and emotions so they work together as a unified whole. Using this approach will make a significant difference in your life.

In holistic health, we also recognize, work with, and see and feel the energy fields or auras. These consist of the etheric body, closely related to the physical form, the emotional body, the mental body, and the spiritual body. These energy fields can be photographed, seen, and felt as distinct, yet sometimes overlapping layers. The aura is made up of different colors, a little like a rainbow.

From the visual pattern of lighter and darker areas or from the way the energy feels, practitioners are able to detect areas of energy imbalance. This gives them additional information about how best to help clients. More darkness or density in a specific energy field can indicate that a health concern may be primarily related to emotional or spiritual factors, for example. Often when I tell a client that her physical concern seems to be related to emotions, she says, "I'm not surprised."

As life happens, our energy field shifts, sometimes changing minute by minute.

If you could see or feel the energy field around the body, you'd know how innerconnected all those layers are. What happens in one layer of the aura affects the others. What happens to one part of the body affects other parts of the body as well as the entire energy system of the universe.

As life happens, our energy field shifts, sometimes changing minute by minute. If we become angry, our energy field will shift, often becoming darker and more congested. If we're feeling intense love or peace, our aura may be brighter, with more intense colors. When we are very focused on thought, our energy field may have more yellow in it.

When we have experiences that cause us to doubt, be less trusting, and feel more alone and separate, the spiritual layers of the aura change. The energy becomes denser and more out of balance with the others. If we aren't able to release that energy on our own, the energy flow at the other layers, mental, emotional, and etheric, will also become more congested, with reduced flow.

Eventually that impeded flow will result in symptoms in the physical body. Without any intervention to release, clear, and balance the energy, the symptoms may lead to a diagnosis from the doctor, medication, and, possibly, a reduced quality of life.

Tiger Tale #4
Slow Flow

Think of the restricted energy flow as a plumbing problem. At first, you'll have a very good flow of water at the kitchen faucet. Gradually you may begin noticing a slightly reduced flow, but it's not a significant problem so you ignore it. As it slows down even more, you start giving it more attention. There must be something wrong. Maybe there's a leak some-where. Maybe a part is wearing out or something is blocking the flow.

If you're feeling competent and self-assured, you may get out some tools and start loosening parts and taking a closer look (after turning off the water supply, of course). Perhaps you'll discover sand and other debris in the filter at the end of the faucet. You clean it out and make a note to check it more often.

If you ignore the problem until you have almost no flow left and are unable to use the sink any more, you may decide to call a plumber. The plumber finds the filter is totally blocked. Furthermore, the extra pressure has caused the pipes underneath the sink to leak. The water is ruining the bottom of the cabinet and the wall and floor below. Now you need lots of repair work. You call in other specialists to help repair the damage. What could have been a small problem has become a big one because it was ignored too long.

Have you been ignoring your tiger too long? Now is the best time to start tuning in to the subtle guidance of your tiger. Listening will help you deal with challenging life experiences more easily.

Most allopathic medicine works primarily with physical problems and not with the body's energy system. The imbalances and restrictions in the energy flow in the early stages go undetected. When the health condition becomes severe enough, physicians usually recommend drugs or surgery.

Often years after surgery or severe accidents, people are still suffering from extreme pain and other symptoms. After one to three sessions of energy therapy with the client, the ongoing symptoms usually are gone completely or are much better.

Lyle's Story

Lyle was one of these clients. We first met at an introductory class I was teaching on energy medicine and pain relief in a local health food store. I demonstrated one of the techniques on Lyle. I found an area of extreme imbalance in his energy that corresponded to the area of his greatest pain. I worked with him for about five minutes.

Often clearing and **balancing** *the energy relieves the pain.*

After the class, Lyle came up to me to tell me he wanted to make an appointment. He continued by saying, "This is the first time I've had any relief from the pain in over five years since my accident."

When Lyle came for his first Healing Touch session, he related this story. "I was driving down the highway when I saw an accident. I stopped and got out to help. A truck came by going about sixty miles an hour, hit me, and threw me into the ditch. I was knocked unconscious. I had a lot of injuries—broken ribs, tailbone and vertebrae, closed head injuries, and lots of pain."

"I got good medical care including physical therapy and lots of time in rehab. I had to quit going to school because I couldn't comprehend what I read. Physically I'm very limited because I have so much pain when I move."

I did a lot of work to clear and balance the energy in the layers of the aura around his body. I held my hands where the energy felt very congested, especially at his back, chest, and head. By the end of the session Lyle said the pain was almost totally gone. In his case, the physical body had repaired itself, but the energy body still needed to be worked with.

A couple of sessions later, Lyle was complaining of some pain in his chest and back. I asked him what he had been doing. Lyle replied, "Driving fence posts manually. I had to reach up above my head to pound them into the ground." I couldn't help but smile as I gently scolded and teased him about taking on such a physically demanding task, and started working to relieve the pain.

By our fourth session, Lyle was back in school and doing well. He was also helping a local politician manage her campaign.

You may know someone who has had a body part removed. Often the person experiences pain in the missing area such as a foot. It's sometimes referred to as "phantom pain." Lyle's pain was due to an injury. In both cases, the pain is related to an imbalance in the energy system. Often clearing and balancing the energy relieves the pain.

Other factors can account for different kinds of pain and discomfort. If your life feels out of balance and painful, you may be under lots of stress and constantly juggling schedules, finances, work, children, relationships, and time constraints. You may find that as you try to balance home and job responsibilities, you discover there's no time left just for you.

Joy's Story
Balancing Act

At one time in my life, I felt the same way. I was running all the time, working hard with long hours, giving to others, but not receiving easily and doing very little just for myself. I was a whiz at analyzing, synthesizing, researching, and planning. Even though I was a very sensitive person, very few of my choices, whether job-related or personal, were made based on what I sensed was best for me.

Following the rules, using logic and reasoning, being fair, meeting expectations (mine and others), and getting the job done well were my priorities at work. Personally, my focus was primarily on recovering from the workweek, doing household tasks and errands, and getting ready to start another week. I was looking forward to the day I could retire.

All of that changed rather abruptly and dramatically. My marriage of nearly thirty years ended. My rapidly declining health made it impossible for me to work at all. Now that really got my attention. Something was definitely not working in my life (besides me).

As I think about it now, I realize it was the balance that was gone. Much of the joy was missing. I wasn't feeling very happy or appreciated.

Think about your story. How happy and peaceful are you now? What are you doing to take care of yourself?

Balance is important in every aspect of your life. Just because you may be surviving a stressful, hectic life style doesn't mean it's desirable. Are you just going to settle, or do you want to feel more joy and peace now?

What kind of message are you giving your children and others you care about? You may feel too busy, tired, and stressed to spend time with the significant people in your life and truly enjoy it. Perhaps there's something you'd really like to do but just haven't found the time or money for. When are you going to start doing what you really want to do with your life? If you wait, it may be too late. As the saying goes, "Tomorrow never comes."

When we continue listening exclusively to our mind, we're not as likely to make the changes we'd like to see. Our mind fuels our emotions. Emotions strongly influence our decisions. Fears, doubts, and rationalizations take over.

The mind and emotions affect the body. Sooner or later we'll begin having more physical symptoms or more emotional ups and downs. When we experience more severe symptoms, we usually take some action. We may or may not associate the way we feel physically with what we're thinking and feeling or how our spiritual health is doing.

Joy's Story
Trash Guilt Trip

Here's a personal example of the powerful relationship between body, mind, and spirit. One morning just before my trash was due to be picked up, I bent over to pick up an empty box to add to the trash at the curb. As I started to straighten up, my back muscles seized up; suddenly I was in severe pain.

I was amazed. The empty box was very light. My back had not been hurting. "What just happened here?" I asked myself. The answer came very quickly. I was feeling guilty because I knew my partner did not like throwing away "perfectly good" boxes no matter how many we had already.

I mentally and emotionally released the feeling of guilt and assured myself that I no longer needed the pain as a punishment for doing a "bad" thing. The pain lessened immediately and disappeared gradually within an hour or so.

The old pattern was to get severe back pain, often for no apparent reason. Then it lasted for weeks or sometimes months. Now I had just learned how easily my mind can cause pain and also, how easily it can release it. This was a very empowering moment for me.

What is your spirit telling you? It may be encouraging you to listen, trust, and believe you can have what you want: joy, peace, love, and more. If you're listening and willing to trust and follow, you'll be guided step by step. Mind, body, and spirit all need to be in alignment for you to feel and be at peace.

You can use your mind as a helpful tool. Remember to reexamine your beliefs, patterns, and practices. Think about what have you been doing that has seemed so important and really isn't.

Set your priorities. Is it more important to make another business call or to go for a quiet walk or a bicycle ride? Is it more important to take on a volunteer leadership role or use the time for self-care or family fun?

How do you define important? Choose what it means to you. Consider that a part of the definition may be about balance. Look at what feels out of balance in your life.

Consider whether it's more important to continue with your stressful, higher-paying position or to look for one not so stressful even if it pays a little less. You may find you'll actually save money on health care, child care, and transportation costs in a new job. Perhaps you can work from your home several days a week. Can you work fewer hours and make a good income if you focus on that?

What is your **spirit** *telling you?*

Another way of looking at balancing and connecting body, mind, and spirit is to look at the differences between how our right- and left-brain see and process information. The left-brain is the analytical, reasoning, planning, calculating part of the brain. It is often referred to as the male side. The left-brain controls the right side of the body.

Pain or other symptoms on the right side may relate to a constriction in the energy related to left-brain functions. Conversely, the right-brain controls the left side of the body. It's given credit for the intuitive, trusting, knowing, creative part of us. The right-brain is associated with feminine energy.

Children, artists, musicians, writers, and other creative people tend to use their right-brain more than other people. Women tend to connect more easily with their right-brain abilities than men. Engineers, doctors, mathematicians, and computer specialists are examples of occupations requiring a high degree of left-brain processing skills. More men tend to use their left-brain almost to the exclusion of their right-brain. Many women are also left-brain dominant; some men are right-brain dominant.

Ideally, all of us will become perfectly balanced between the left- and right-brain and male and female energies. Men and women alike have both male and female qualities and tendencies. Let's appreciate the similarities and celebrate the differences among all people.

For instance, as women we tend to multi-task very well. We can talk on the phone, prepare a bank deposit, help a customer, and sign for a package delivery pretty much all at the same time. Men, you generally focus on one thing at a time and don't seem to be able to multi-task as well. We women wonder why men can't do what we can do. Men, you wonder why women flit from one thing to another.

It's not that one thing is wrong and the other is right. Both have a place. However, as a recovering master multi-tasker, I have to say that I see a definite advantage to the typical male approach. Focusing on one thing at a time actually keeps you more fully in the moment and allows you to give your undivided attention to whatever you are doing. Start increasing your awareness of the multitude of ways you can support and complement each other in your day-to-day experiences.

Ross' Story

Ross was a client who was very aware of the interconnection of body, mind, and spirit. He came to me initially for help in relieving anxiety, improving his focus, and pacing himself better with his work. He also had some minor physical symptoms.

During the first session with Ross, I discovered an imbalance in his energy system. The energy at his upper chakras, or energy centers in the body, was out of balance with the lower chakras. The energy was going in two different directions. I intuited that Ross was struggling with a lot of conflict.

"It seems that your upper chakras, which relate to intuition, using your power, and spiritual guidance, are telling you one thing," I told Ross. "Your lower chakras, which relate more to fear, relationships, and physical well-being, are resisting that guidance. The anxiety may be, in part, related to the conflict you're feeling. You already know what to do."

Ross replied, "I have known of a new direction in my work and have resisted making a change due to my insecurity about the unknown and the fear of not being able to support my family. The information you shared is right on. I know it's time to change and release the fear."

You already **know** *what to do.*

I cleared and balanced the energy in his body and energy field. I encouraged Ross to follow his intuition, which was already fairly strong, and to trust his guidance. I also suggested a breathing technique to use. I asked him to feel the energy in his body related to different choices he was considering one at a time. This method helps improve the balance between body, mind, spirit, and emotions.

In this case, Ross already knew at a spiritual, intuitive level what he was being guided to do. His mind had been resisting it. Emotionally, Ross was feeling fear and anxiety. Physically, he was not sleeping well and was experiencing some pain. Once Ross stopped resisting his guidance, the mental, emotional, and physical energy bodies became smoother and calmer.

Donna's Story

Donna was struggling with her relationship with her husband. We talked about it each time she came to see me. I worked with her to release the congested energy and balance it.

Donna continued to feel stressed and uncertain about what to do. She was tired and confused and felt like she was on an emotional roller coaster. I suggested Donna take some time to connect with that inner place of knowing, and see what her guidance told her. We talked about ways for her to gain more clarity.

I told Donna when she got a clear message to follow it. She subsequently got greater clarity and acted on it. When I saw Donna the next time, she was "sparkling" and beaming. "I feel so free and peaceful." Donna continues to feel happy with the course of action she has chosen.

Both Ross and Donna found that when they let their minds and emotions take over, they felt more and more confused, anxious, and emotionally unsettled. When they connected with and listened to their spiritual guidance, they got more clarity, acted on it with less fear, and felt greater freedom and peace.

You, too, can bring your body, mind, and spirit into harmony. Feel the signals and signs from your body; see how they relate to what is happening in your mind and life experiences. Pay attention to what your mind is telling you and what you and others are saying. Listen to what your heart is saying. All of them have important messages for you. Follow your inner knowing.

You, too, can bring your body, mind, and spirit into harmony.

Empowerment Guide

- Complementary health care practitioners actively focus on helping you balance and connect the body, mind, and spirit.
- Layers of the energy field around the body correspond to the body's emotions, mind, and spirit. They can be used for early detection of energy imbalances in the body.

- Pain and other symptoms can often be alleviated, even years after an accident or surgery, by clearing, balancing, and connecting the energy system.

- Gaining control of your life and making what's really important a priority will help you become more balanced, peaceful, and joyful.

- Relying primarily on your mind and emotions can keep you feeling trapped, stressed, confused, and unhappy. This often leads to pain and other physical symptoms and illness.

- We each affect everything and everyone else, so choose your thoughts, actions, and surroundings wisely.

- Valuing and using both our left- and right-brained abilities can lead to inner and outer balance.

- Following the spirit within will help you connect body, mind, and spirit in a peaceful, joyful way.

Action Guide

Affirmations:

I am continually aware of the body, mind, spirit connection and use that to help me make adjustments in what I think, say, and do.

I easily find ways to create greater peace and harmony in my life.

Energy Technique:

If you feel out of sorts or your energy seems out of balance, tap on the thymus (high heart area) just above the heart for about fifteen seconds. Apply gentle pressure just below your collarbone and about a hand's width to the right of the center of your body. When you have located the correct place, it most likely will be tender. Repeat on the left side.

Inner Connecting: Tiger Spirit

Get into a comfortable position. Take three deep breaths, exhaling any stress and tension you may feel. Now, starting with your feet and moving slowly up your body: knees, upper legs, hips, and beyond, notice any areas that feel especially tight or uncomfortable.

Choose one area to work with. Breathe into it with your full attention. Now ask yourself when you first noticed discomfort or imbalance in this area. What was going on in your life? Who were you with? What were you thinking or talking about? What relationship is there between them? Ask for additional insight from the spirit of the tiger within. What changes can you make that will help you feel more relaxed and balanced?

Send loving energy to this area and any other areas of tension. When they feel calm and full of love, slowly take three deep breaths and begin bringing your attention back to the space around you.

Essential Oils:

German Blue Chamomile

- German Blue Chamomile improves and supports a variety of physical conditions, promotes emotional balance, and soothes and clears the mind, leading to greater peace. Dilute one drop of oil in one teaspoon of honey or four ounces of liquid and ingest or apply the oil topically on a specific area of concern or diffuse into the air.

More Steps to Tiger Spirit:

- Look for creative ways to bring your life into balance and harmony.

- Reexamine how you're using your time. Prioritize your activities. Which are the most rewarding, fulfilling, or necessary? Listen to your guidance. Choose which things you can eliminate or minimize to make more time to nurture and energize yourself and make room for exciting new ventures.

- Start paying attention to the relationship between your body, mind, and spirit. Is the pain or loss of energy you just began noticing related to what you've been thinking about or feeling recently? Are you experiencing a symptom that isn't responding to treatment as the doctors expected? If so, look for a mental, emotional, or spiritual connection and seek help for releasing and balancing that energy.

Healing Guide

How are you doing with balancing your life's activities? Peace and joy will come to you more easily if you first connect with your spiritual knowing, your inner tiger. Then use body and mind to support and assist you in following that knowing.

Abundance is knowing
that when we give from
a loving, compassionate
heart, we always

receive

more than we give.

CHAPTER SIX

Abundance, Tiger Style

Manifesting Your Desires

WHAT IS YOUR BODY, MIND, SPIRIT association with abundance? What do you think of when you think of abundance? Your body and spirit may have a different sense of abundance.

Connecting with abundance is the sixth path on the journey. Abundance means many things to many people. You may think of it as money or financial status. You may see abundance as that which allows you to do what you want to do. You may think of it as having adequate food, clothing, or shelter.

Ultimately, abundance is not about money, power, material goods, or relationships with others. Abundance is actually a state of being and of belief. It's a belief that there's always enough. Tiger abundance is giving from the heart. Tiger abundance is trusting in the power of love and peace. Tiger abundance is knowing that when we give from a loving, compassionate heart, we always receive more than we give.

Our personal attitude about abundance actually affects the flow of energy coming and going to and from us. Have you thought of abundance only as inflow, or have you also seen it as outflow? Abundance is like a two-way street or a superhighway. Traffic flows both ways, coming and going, up and down, and in and out.

If you have been visualizing only a one-way street to your house, let go of that image now. Seeing abundance only as what you have, what you don't have, and what you want is very restrictive. Holding onto everything you have and living in fear of not having enough, slows the flow.

Tiger Tale #5
Water, Water Everywhere

Think of abundance as a steady stream of water flowing to and from your house. It's fresh, sparkling, and life-sustaining. Then you start thinking, "What if this stream dried up? What would I do for water?" So you develop a plan to keep from running out of water.

You fill every container you can find with this wonderful water. You store the containers in a spare bedroom. Then you decide this might not be enough, so you purchase more and more containers. You fill each one and store them inside your house so they'll be safe.

Your house becomes so full of containers, barrels, buckets, and bathtubs filled with water that you can't move around. You can't find anything else or enjoy your normal activities due to lack of space. You don't want to use any of the water you stored for cleaning, bathing, and drinking because you might need it later.

> Giving increases the flow of energy and helps manifest more of what you want.

Eventually you get depressed, your health starts failing, and the water stored in the containers stagnates. The flow of energy and abundance has nearly stopped. It's all around you, but you aren't able to access it.

You may say, "I scrimp and save and do without, and still there's never enough." Fear has slowed the flow of abundance. Now all you see and feel is lack. Your house, which once seemed spacious, now feels much too small. You no longer remember that the fresh stream of water is running next to your house, and you can access it at any time.

Instead of hoarding water, you could have chosen to trust that the water would continue to flow. You also could have shared the water with others or nourished the plants and yourself. You could have offered to help carry water for others farther from the stream or for those less physically able. Giving increases the flow of energy and helps manifest more of what you want.

Doug's Story

I know a man, Doug, who is a collector. He's not your typical collector. He doesn't go out looking for interesting, unusual, valuable, or fun things. He doesn't decide what he wants and then begin focusing on it.

Doug's collectibles usually come home with him from grocery stores, discount stores, delivery services, or the mailbox. In practice, this shows up as jars and bottles of all sizes and shapes gracing his kitchen counters and the top of the refrigerator. He has a massive collection of baby food jars even though he's now a senior citizen. Paper bags, plastic bags, twist ties, empty cans, and boxes all vie for space in the kitchen, garage, stairways, furniture, and floors. Styrofoam peanuts abound. Junk mail has a place of honor on tabletops and chair seats.

Doug often says, "I'm running out of room to put things." He doesn't want anyone to come to his big, beautiful house because of all the "stuff" he has collected. I suggested an easy solution to this dilemma…several boxes of large trash bags. I don't think he was either amused or interested.

What's behind this behavior? Doug says, "You never know when you might need something." The catch to that is you have to be able to find it first.

The primary reasons for this kind of collecting are fear and lack of trust. It comes from feeling there won't be enough. "I need to save this. If

I throw it away, I might not be able to get another one when I need it." As with the first example, Doug's belief in not having enough slows the flow of abundance.

Fear is also what caused people to panic during the Great Depression of the 1930s. People perceived and feared lack. Because of their beliefs, thoughts, and feelings, they acted in a way that exacerbated the concept of lack: selling stocks, withdrawing funds from banks, hoarding, and not spending.

In actuality, there was no shortage. In the United States, more grain was stored for future use than ever before. If people had focused on what they really wanted and put energy into creating that, there would have been no "real" loss.

This idea of saving for a rainy day doesn't serve us well. I'm not talking about saving for college expenses or a down payment or having a reasonable cushion for extra expenses in your bank account. I'm referring to hoarding out of fear of what might happen or fear of lack.

What you really want to create is an attitude of plenty and of abundance.

This rainy-day kind of thinking actually contributes to making it rain. It gives energy to creating the exact opposite of what you want. Your focus is on lack: "What if there isn't enough?" What you really want to create is an attitude of plenty and of abundance.

You may feel that you aren't able to connect with abundance. You may feel that you've tried manifesting before, and it never works for you. You may ask, "What am I doing wrong?" Here are some general guidelines to consider.

First of all, let's be certain you're not confusing manifestation with wishful thinking. Wishful thinking is having thoughts with no belief, passion, feeling, or action.

Second, let's go back to that body, mind, spirit connection we spoke of earlier. All three of these areas are essential in creating what you desire along with the emotional energy to support them. They work synergistically. If one element is missing, you may not manifest what you really want. In fact, you may be creating the opposite of what you desire.

Actually, we don't create abundance. It already exists everywhere, in and around everything and everyone. We tap into it by believing abundance is always with us and always available to us. We manifest from abundance, the vast potentiality that is.

> *We manifest from* **abundance,** *the vast potentiality that is.*

One way to think of manifesting is as an equilateral triangle. Now write body, mind, or spirit at each of the three corners. Spirit represents passion, guidance, and desire. Mind represents belief and thoughts. The body takes action and does what needs to be done in the outer world. What you are creating goes in the center. Emotions tie all the sides or parts together.

Let's look at manifesting another way as outlined below:

- Desire — What is your passion? Think of it as the voice of guidance. Dare to dream big.

- Believe — Believe and trust in yourself and your ability to create. Believe you can create what you want. Know Spirit is always supporting you.

- See — Visualize what you want. You must be able to see it to create it.

- Feel — Feel your emotions, inner excitement, and enthusiasm.

- Act — Act as if it's happening now. When an opportunity arises or you get an impulse or intuitive flash, trust it and act on it. Take steps to achieve it. Do what it takes to create your dream.

- Focus — Focus your thoughts, attention, emotions, and actions on what you want, day-by-day and moment-by-moment. Be persistent in pursuing your vision.

Remember to give gratitude for what you have and for what is. Being grateful for the "little" things as well as the "big" things helps create more of what you desire. Share your abundance: skills, time, energy, money, knowledge, and other resources. Also be open to receiving abundance.

If you think you've been following these but without success, look at these common interference patterns.

- Negativity — This is based on limiting beliefs from past experiences projected into the present and the future. "This is what I want but ..."
- Non-deserving attitude — "Who do I think I am, expecting *that* will happen? I don't deserve anything that good."
- Non-belief — "This is what I'd like, but I don't believe it's possible. No one could *really* do that."
- Inconsistency — You say one thing and do another. You see and think the opposite of what you really want. The message you're sending to Spirit is unclear.
- Omission — One of the essential elements is missing: desire, passion, belief, thoughts, emotions, or action.
- Limited focus — You start out with high energy and focus, but you soon get busier with life activities and expend little or no effort manifesting what you desire.

In a football game, using these patterns would be like having so much interference the receiver can't complete the reception and reach the goal.

More of Brenda's Story

The following story comes from my work with Brenda, a client whom you met earlier. In this session, I found the energy at Brenda's left arm was not flowing well. I asked her if her arm had been bothering her lately. She said, "Yes. Actually both of my arms have been feeling strange lately." As I continued doing energy work to improve the energy flow in her arms, I intuited that this was not about what was happening on the physical level. It seemed more emotional or spiritual.

"Your arms are about holding things and embracing," I said. "They also give us messages about implementing change and going in a new direction. I sense that you are to share your wisdom with others from a place of empowerment. Somehow, it seems, you may be blocking that."

Brenda said, "Well, I have thought about teaching classes. I'd like to teach one on one, working with bullies like my mom, but I'm *afraid* of attracting the "wrong people.""

"Let's talk about that," I suggested. "It's so important to watch our thoughts. We can create what we don't want just as easily as what we *do* want. Every time you think of what you *don't* want, you give energy to it, which helps attract it to you."

"So," I continued, "switch to thinking of what you want. See it, feel it, believe it, talk about it. That will bring energy to what you *do* want. Trust that you'll know the right time to offer the class and that the right people will be there."

"Thanks," Brenda responded. "That helps a lot." At that moment the restricted energy flow at her arms released.

More of Ross' Story

Here's another story about Ross, whom you met in the last chapter. We have focused on helping him get "unstuck" related to his work and moving in a new direction. We did some energetic emotional release techniques (EER) and other energy-balancing work. Ross was able to feel the flow of energy in his body. His awareness of how he was resisting and blocking his guidance increased. I pointed out to Ross that it appeared he was focusing on what he didn't want: stuckness.

I asked Ross to focus on his breath and feel the effect of different options on his body, as I described in Chapter Five. I suggested just following the guidance he has been given for the next step. We talked about trusting in the flow of energy and not needing to know the whole, detailed plan.

At the beginning of his next session, Ross shared that a lot had happened since he saw me a couple weeks ago. He had a dream with a very vivid symbol that he understood well due to his profession. It consisted of two overlapping circles. In the common area in the center, Ross saw a squiggly symbol for resistance. He felt the dream showed him how he had been resisting change.

Several days later Ross also got an intuitive message that said, "Look beyond." He interpreted that to mean that he needed to look beyond what he was seeing and doing currently and make some changes. Finally, a man who works in the same office building offered Ross a new business opportunity in his area of expertise that would be less stressful and more rewarding. It was exactly what Ross had in mind even though the initial income was uncertain. He was excited about making some changes.

The Law of Attraction (LOA) states that like attracts like. What we think about is what we get. If we think about what we don't want, we'll get more of what we don't want. If we think we're stuck, then we'll stay stuck because that's what our focus is. That's where our energy is going. If we focus our attention on illness, we'll attract more illness. If we focus on health, we'll attract health.

Just like magnets attract, we become and attract what we think and feel. Thoughts have an energetic frequency that radiates out from us and attracts what we sent out. Think of the body, mind, and spirit as a powerful magnet that sends out and attracts certain energies to us according to what we desire, think, feel, and do. This includes friends, opportunities, work, experiences, and more.

Using an Internet dating service has become a popular and effective way to draw new people to you. When you decide to do this, you already have the intent to match up with someone who has similar interests, beliefs, and intent. You send out that energy, information, and message. You follow up with appropriate action: checking your e-mail, reading information sent to you, sensing which ones are the best matches for you, and responding accordingly.

If you're not getting positive results, you may have some emotional energy or negative beliefs about yourself and your ability to be successful that are getting in the way. You may have a sense of unworthiness or low self-esteem. You may be focusing on what you don't want.

"I don't want anyone fat, ugly, lazy, uninteresting ..." In this example, where is your focus? These thoughts and feelings interfere with attaining the outcome you desire. Change your focus, and you change the outcome. For example: "I desire someone who is physically attractive and energetic and has many interests and hobbies."

Change your focus, and you **change** *the outcome.*

The Law of Attraction is a very powerful force in our universe. However, other factors also come into play in our lives. For example, what is your soul's mission or your divine purpose? Are you here for a specific purpose or just to experience flowing with what is? How well are you able to do this? Do you resist and rebel against everything that is not going the way you envisioned? Can you just allow it to *be,* while peacefully following your guidance to show you the next step?

If you desire something that is totally beyond your physical capabilities, then it may not happen. If you're setting out to acquire a billion dollars, you may be disappointed. Striving for more material or worldly things may not bring you happiness. This is especially true if your goal is to attain greater influence or control over people or if it isn't congruent with bringing you inner peace.

More of Francine's Story

Francine, whom you met earlier, was working with me to relieve pain and a rash on her neck and upper chest. It was related to emotional and spiritual congestion in her energy field. The throat area relates to communication; not speaking up or speaking your truth.

Francine wanted to find a new job but hadn't taken any action yet. She was not sure she'd get another one. We talked about being positive and putting energy into what she wanted.

At the next session, Francine shared the following experience with me. She had updated her résumé and written a letter of introduction. While she was doing this, Francine visualized herself getting her ideal job. She had very positive feelings while preparing the letters for mailing. She put them altogether in one pile, held her hands over them, and prayed. Finally, Francine let go of the outcome and trusted Spirit to bring her ideal job to her.

A few days later John, a recipient of one of her letters, called, said he liked what she had to say, and set up an interview with her. After the interview, John told Francine the job was hers. He was planning to build a new facility that would be ready in a few months. John told Francine she could set it up the way she wanted and would be the lead person in her area of responsibility.

Francine was ecstatic. She loved John's ideas and energy and had a good feeling about her new boss.

What do you want? Use your power, and let your thoughts, emotions, beliefs, visualizations, and actions create that. You can have what you truly desire if you'll give up the belief that you can't have it.

You may find you have the desire and passion for creating what you want, but you get hung up at the belief step. To help you move past this, ask yourself this question. "If I didn't believe what I desired was impossible, what would I do?"

You will most likely come up with an answer for this question. When you do, just take the next step as you would if you really believed it were possible. Then, what would you do next if you believed it were possible? Take that step also.

As you continue taking steps to achieve your dream, you'll feel excitement growing. You will see yourself being joyful and successful, and you'll notice changes in yourself. Almost before you realize it, your belief will have shifted. You'll be well into creating what you want.

Joy's Story
Manifesting Tables

Here's a simple example from my experience. I really wanted a massage table to use in my work when I was first starting my practice. I wanted to get a used table in good condition at a reasonable price. Most people I talked to in related businesses said, "Oh, you'll never find a used table. They go so quickly no one ever lists them for sale."

Disappointed and about ready to give up on getting what I wanted, I talked to my coach. She told me to ignore what I had been told. She said, "Just set your intent. Be specific about what you want, including the timeframe and the price. Take action to get the word out, and trust Spirit do the rest.

I wrote out a notice of what I wanted on index cards. I posted them on the bulletin boards at two local health food stores. A week later I attended a seminar out of town. When I stopped at a health food store to get something to eat, I noticed a newspaper lying on top of the other stack of papers. It was folded open to the miscellaneous section of the want ads. I decided to pick it up and look at it. The ad listing a massage table for sale practically jumped off the page at me. I purchased that table before I left for home.

The next day I received a call from a woman who had seen my notice posted at a health food store. I bought the table she had for sale even though I already had one. Two days after arriving home, I received a call from a man who also had a table for sale. I thanked him and told him I had just purchased two massage tables.

So I not only found one used massage table, but three. Obviously, if I had continued to believe what I wanted was impossible, I would not even have tried to find a used table.

Be careful what you think because that's what you may get. If you find yourself thinking of what you don't want, observe what you're doing and gently shift your thoughts or actions to what you *do* want. Increasingly, your awareness of how you've been creating more of what you *don't* want will help you keep your thoughts more focused on manifesting what you *do* want.

Imagine yourself as an artist painting a picture of your life just the way you want it. Take your time and use colors and shapes you like. Experiment with different options. Try a new technique or pattern. Relax and have fun with it.

Since you are constantly creating, why not put your energy into creating peace, joy, and love? Now you know what it takes. It's not difficult. Be willing to let go of any negative beliefs, thoughts, and visualizations and replace them with positive ones. Remember...you are the creator of the world you see and experience.

Remember ... you are the **creator** *of the world you see and experience.*

Empowerment Guide

- Hoarding slows the flow of abundance.

- Saving for a rainy day gives energy to manifesting the opposite of what we want: a time of lack, depression, and being down and out.

- Abundance is everywhere; is constant and inexhaustible. It's always available to us. There is no lack.

- Believe in yourself and the power of positive thoughts and actions.

- Our thoughts create our world. Think and feel what you *do* want instead of what you *don't* want.

- Passion is empowering.

- Manifesting what we desire requires positive, focused attention on body, mind, spirit, and emotions.

- Steps to manifestation include: desiring, believing, seeing, feeling, acting, focusing, giving, and receiving.

- Giving gratitude daily, for what we have and for what is, creates more to be grateful for.

Action Guide

Affirmations:

I attract whatever I desire, believe in, and focus on: money, health, people, connections, peace, and joy. (Substitute one or more of your own instead.)

I draw to me more of what I give gratitude for.

Energy Technique:

Place one hand at your solar plexus, your power center in the middle of your body beneath your ribs, and one hand over your heart. Hold both these areas until they feel peaceful, calm, and balanced. Focus your intent for creating what you want at your heart center. Feel the energy increasing and building momentum.

Now take your attention to your solar plexus. Feel the power within you becoming focused in this area. Bring that energy up to your heart and combine it with your heart's desire, your thoughts, feelings, and emotions. Feel and know how powerful you are. Give gratitude for the blessings in your life.

Relax your hands when it feels right to you. Smile and carry this positive, powerful feeling with you as you continue creating.

Inner Connecting: Tiger Flow

Get into a quiet space and a comfortable position. Close your eyes. Focus on your breath and slow your breathing. Think of the air you're breathing as a field of limitless possibilities flowing in and out with each breath. Notice all the colors in this field. Find your favorite ones and breathe them in and out, letting them fill your body and energy field around your body with color.

Now focus your attention on the field of possibilities again. It's filled with feelings and emotions. Find the ones you're most attracted to and pull them into your energy field with your breath and your intent.

Once again, return to this expanded field of potentiality. Somewhere in this field is your passion, your "burning" desire. Anything you could ever want, dare to hope for or visualize, and more, is in this vastness. You'll most likely be attracted to it easily and effortlessly. If you haven't found it yet, then attract one with your imagination. What does it look like, and how does it feel? Do any thoughts, words, or messages come to you from deep inside, from that place of heart-knowing? Listen carefully. Connect with your passion deeply and completely.

Now place that passion within into a flower you are drawn to from that field of possibilities. Make the flower one of your favorite colors. Add the feelings and emotions you were attracted to before. Infuse any thoughts, words, or messages that came to you about your passion.

With your hands, slowly bring the passion-filled flower to your heart and gently place it inside. Here it will be nurtured and grow into what you desire. As you focus your attention on it, bring your awareness back to your body and the space around you. Take three deep breaths and open your eyes when you're ready.

Note: You may choose to write down any impressions, messages, significant words, or thoughts that came to you during the inner connecting. As you repeat this meditation, you may find that, even though you may be focusing on the same passion each time, your experience may be different with different thoughts, words, inspirations, or visualizations.

Essential Oils:

Myrrh and Geranium

- Myrrh promotes spiritual awareness and is uplifting. It helps open our hearts and minds to receiving. Apply on the bottom of your feet, on the area of concern, or diffuse into the air.

- Geranium helps balance emotions, lift the spirit, and promote peace and hope. Use in the same manner as for Myrrh above.

More Steps to Tiger Flow

- Express heartfelt gratitude for every experience, every person, and every day whether it's filled with sunshine or rain. We need *both* to grow and be healthy.

- Continue to believe in your vision. Work toward this vision for as long as it takes.

- Think and speak about what makes you feel good and energizes you and what you'd like more of. Focus on how you can change your life instead of having a "woe is me" attitude.

- Write down the change you want to see and be and focus on creating that.

- Find pictures, words, and sayings that represent your vision, and attach them to a bulletin board or poster board. Use ones that make you smile, feel good, and excite you. Look at the board often and feel the energy of what you are manifesting.

- Focus on what you want moment by moment while giving thanks for it and all that is.

- Journal every day about what you're grateful for. Include the "little" things as well as the more significant ones, e.g. the wonderful feeling of the sun warming your body and spirit, making a new friend, or receiving an unexpected refund check in the mail.

Healing Guide

Abundance is more than creating material goods, wealth, and opportunity. It's about finding ways to bring joy and peace into your life. It's about appreciating and honoring everything that's part of your life and your experiences. It's about being okay with who you are, just as you are. Can you allow others to be who they are and to see the world as they choose? Use your power to create what you desire at a deep level. Allow All That Is, however it shows up in your life.

The ability to feel
and extend love comes
from a sense of

oneness

with all people and
all things.

CHAPTER SEVEN

The **Tiger** and the **Team**

Creating Unity

THE SEVENTH PATH ON THE JOURNEY of healing and empowerment is feeling the oneness of All That Is. Now that you are aware you can create more of what you want and less of what you don't want, why on earth would you create separateness? Why would you create something separate from yourself that you can compare, judge, criticize, and attack? Then you can expect to receive the same in return. This sounds crazy. Well, you didn't...at least your true self didn't.

Instead, it is the ego self that sees us as separate from everything and everyone else, including God or Spirit. By feeling separate, we can blame, worry, and stress out because life, our job, or our finances aren't following our expectations. We say, "I thought I planned everything so well. This wasn't supposed to happen. Now what am I going to do?" We're unhappy, disappointed, and ready to kick or whip the first thing or person who gets in our way...or totally retreat.

The ego is strengthened and fed by both misfortune and fortune. If our lives are going poorly for us, the ego will look for a scapegoat, a reason for our lack of progress or success. It will make excuses, attack self and others and say, "See I told you so. You never should have ..."

The ego feeds on fear, greed, guilt, and dissatisfaction. It is fueled by stress, busyness, and worry. Identifying with the ego defines "self" in terms of what we do, like, have, status in life, physical descriptors, what others think of us, mental and creative abilities, and so forth.

If things are going well for us, the ego makes comparisons with other people and judges them. The ego may say things like, "I sure am glad I'm smarter than most people. I wouldn't want to be like my brother-in-law. I don't understand why poor people don't get out and work. They're just lazy." On the flip side, the ego may tell us we're not good enough or we're a failure. Then we may get depressed, discouraged, and disillusioned and turn on ourselves.

Our challenge is to use the ego in a way that supports, inspires, and frees us rather than making us feel alone and unloved.

There's another part of the ego that is often forgotten or overlooked. The ego is also the source of hidden or undeveloped talents, passions, and creativity. So one part of the ego says, "You are better than _____" or "You're not as good as _____." Another aspect says, "You can do anything you desire. Let's try something new."

Our challenge is to use the ego in a way that supports, inspires, and frees us rather than making us feel alone and unloved. Ultimately the ego just is. It really cannot be separated from All That Is.

Very young children are delightful to observe. Initially they have very little restrictive, ego-based thinking or behavior. They seem to flow very easily with what's happening around them. The young ones have few or no inhibitions about commenting on what they observe or doing what feels good.

Scott's Story

One of my fondest memories occurred when my grandson Scott was about three. He was bright, quick, and coordinated. However, certain aspects of soccer confused him.

At one point in the game, Scott got the ball and started dribbling the ball down the field as he had been taught. The coaches were yelling; the parents were shouting. Scott ran and ran, leaving the other young players and the adults far behind. He ran past the other team's goal with the ball just ahead of him and continued running and dribbling, running and dribbling. Most of his three-year-old teammates were oblivious to what was happening; his coach just laughed.

By this time all the spectators, including Grandma, were laughing. His dad ran after him, eventually bringing him and the soccer ball back to the playing field.

This story is short and simple and also illustrates a lack of ego concern. I could say that Scott was following his inner guidance rather than listening to all the separate outer voices trying to influence him. In this case, Scott wasn't unhappy with himself for running the wrong way. He just seemed to be enjoying the experience of running and dribbling, running and dribbling.

If you're not aware, you'll find that the ego works full-time to sap your energy, zap your peace, and trap your joy. However, the ego has no power of its own. It has only the power you give it. You may be wondering how you do that.

Well, when we look to someone or something outside ourselves to tell us who we are or how great or terrible we are, we lose our power. Whenever we make a comparison or a judgment, we weaken our energy and bolster the ego's power.

When we have an almost compulsive desire to understand everything and continue asking "why" and "how" continuously, we are giving up some

of our power. The ego loves these behaviors because by trying to understand life situations and events, we are expressing our need to know. Then
we can judge, evaluate, criticize, and resist. We complain, "It isn't fair.
That shouldn't be."

Patrice's Story

Patrice, a client, is tired, stressed, and constantly seeking answers and
solutions for her physical complaints. She is an example of someone who
has a great need to know, understand, and control what's happening
around her.

Patrice asks many, many questions, often on the same theme. Instead
of "Twenty Questions," it sometimes seems like "One Hundred Questions."
Why? How long? Did you …? When did…? Often the questions seem
designed to determine whether she has been excluded in some way. At
other times it seems she's trying to see if she agrees with what someone
did or how she would have done it differently.

"We are **one** *in Spirit."*

The physical symptoms and behaviors are
related to emotional, mental, and spiritual issues.
Patrice is experiencing a lot of resistance to
letting go of old patterns and fears. Ultimately
she feels abandoned by the world and Spirit. As a
result Patrice has difficulty trusting Spirit, others,
and, of course, her inner knowing. She is seeing and feeling "twoness"
instead of "oneness." It's her against the world instead of being one with it.

Most religions teach that there is one Spirit, one higher consciousness, and that's all there is. They say, "We are one in Spirit." However, in
many religious institutions that truth of oneness is lost in the application
and day-to-day practice.

Too often the message becomes one of hellfire and damnation, of
judgment, political activism, lack of financial support, and being superior

to those of another religion, race, or belief system. It evolves into teachings of fear, separation, guilt, and unworthiness. Unfortunately, the message of love for self and others, unending abundance, being grateful for what is, and acknowledging the perfection of All That Is , is all but lost.

Instead it becomes a message of "twoness," of duality. Are you one of them or one of us? Are you a sinner or a saint (or an aspiring saint)? Messengers, even well-intentioned ones, are sometimes misguided, confused, or obsessed with control. Listen to, and do, what feels right to you and not what others say you should believe or do.

If you were raised with religious dogma, see how this influences your current perception of yourself and your world. You may feel helpless to act or think differently from what you've been taught by religious leaders, parents, family, friends, and life experiences.

If so, remember you can always choose to perceive in a new way, one that helps you feel freer and more empowered. Sift through what you have learned. Be willing to let go of all you've learned and find your own truth.

Pay attention to that **inner knowing.**

Start examining your beliefs. Look for the deeper truth. Notice how you feel when you think about a specific belief. If you feel tense, less peaceful, more helpless, trapped, constricted, confused, or conflicted, it's time to let it go. It isn't congruent with your heart-knowing. If you feel calmer and freer, and more peaceful, joyful, loving, and empowered, that's your tiger within pointing you to the unchanging truth of the oneness. Pay attention to that inner knowing.

The good news is that since you have bought into the concept of duality in your world, you can make another choice. The ego encourages you to compare and evaluate, sort and select, based on who's better, smarter, and nicer. You can stop listening to ego-based thinking. Cease believing the part of the ego that is trying to convince you that everything you see and hear is true.

Instead of seeing yourself and others as separate ego forms, look at them as extensions of yourself, as manifestations of Spirit. To transcend ego-based thinking, focus on connecting with Spirit, the oneness of all there is. The ability to feel and extend love comes from a sense of oneness with all people, plants, and animals rather than feeling separateness.

Melody's Story

Melody, another client, shared the following experience with me that further illustrates the idea of separateness versus oneness.

> *I was at church praying when a young lady asked me to pray for her husband. I was reluctant to do so as I knew a bit of his history, and when I was around him, he just "felt" heavy and dark. The young lady was persistent and would not relent. I sat there asking God to give me the motivation to go pray for her husband because there was nothing in me to do so.*
>
> *Jesus asked me to look at the man again, and suddenly I saw the most beautiful display of purple and blue lights above and around the man that I have ever witnessed. They were moving and felt alive while at the same time a feeling of majestic awesomeness came over me. I heard the Lord say that that's how He sees the man and all of us.*
>
> *In no time I was at the man's side, thanking God for such a magnificent being and the privilege of praying for his need. From that day on, I called him "The Prince of England" since I felt he was royalty, the King's son.*

Just think of how quickly and completely our world would change if everyone could have a similar experience that would shift an individual's perceptions. If people would see others as the beautiful spiritual beings they are instead of as separate ego forms, we would all know the peace of oneness, All That Is.

Do you remember the rainbow bridge of Chapter Four? That bridge not only connects us to Spirit, but it also joins us to every other person, animal, and thing, including the earth. Think of it as an etheric, unseen line of energy connecting everything and everyone.

The earth and everyone on it are part of a giant web of invisible energy particles and waves. A gigantic grid or matrix of energy surrounds the earth. Each person, animal, and thing has an energy field. Everyone is connected through the energy within and around the body. These fields are constantly fluctuating and interacting. Whatever happens to one part of the energy field affects all.

Words, thoughts, and actions have the same effect on the energy matrix that makes up everything in the universe and beyond. When our energy shifts, the energy of everything around us changes. If we're stressed, often others seem to be stressed and anxious too. When we're happier and more peaceful, others feel it and respond differently; usually they're unaware of why they feel better.

Everyone is **connected** *through the energy within and around the body.*

You have very likely felt "spread too thin," scattered or "torn" in two (or more) directions many times. Sometimes it's about being too busy—too many things to do and not enough time. That's when it's very helpful to slow way down and take time to listen to the message of the inner tiger. Yet most people listen to the voice of the ego and try to go faster and faster. Then they wonder what's wrong and why they're not happy.

When we're feeling pulled in two directions, it's usually related to a conflict between the ego's voice and our inner voice. The ego tells us what we should and shouldn't do. It tells us, "It's selfish to take care of yourself first. People will think you don't care about them and you're unreliable." The ego says, "You must work harder, later, and faster. Run, run, run! Stay busy. Being quiet means you're lazy, and it's a big waste of time."

This feeling of being split in two, of having to be in two places at the same time and needing to find the real you is a common human experience.

Remember the old classic television show "To Tell the Truth" where the contestants all claimed to be the same person? Near the end of the show the host asked, "Will the real _____ stand up?

Do you sometimes wonder who the real you is? You can appear to be a different person from one moment to the next. You present different faces or aspects of yourself according to the situation, the people you're with, your emotions, and how you're feeling about yourself. Even a feeling of depression may, in some cases, be related to this split or this yearning for wholeness.

Wholeness is both healing and empowering.

Wholeness is both healing and empowering. Coming from a place of empowerment and healing allows us to be peaceful in the moment as well as being our genuine, authentic self.

The voice of truth deep inside may say that you're tired and being quiet and restful would feel good and help you regain your energy. The message may be, "You can change this. Slow down, listen, and find peace within."

It's quite easy to tell which voice we're hearing. If the message causes us to feel tense, more rushed, more dissatisfied, and unhappier, it's coming from the ego. If we feel calm, loved, and reassured, the voice is that of truth and of Spirit. Which one are you listening to?

Joy's Dream

A recent dream exemplifies this sense of being split in two.

Lacy, a friend and client, appears in my office. As I am talking to her, she splits into two identical bodies so quickly and easily it's difficult to tell exactly how it happened. The bodies seem to be in two different places with two unique personas. One Lacy is much like she usually is: upbeat, talkative, and full of energy. The other Lacy is very quiet, withdrawn, and depressed.

I ask the women in the adjacent room if they've seen the quiet Lacy. They say, "No."

I respond, "We need to find her so I can put her together again." I sense that since she came from one being, we need to find the separate parts and unify them into one. I continue searching for Lacy's missing self with no success.

Then I see examples of two people who are choosing to heal as one couple. Near the end of the dream, two "men" lose their heads, revealing robot bodies. Since they turn out not to be "real," I am free to do what I chose to do.

The message I got from this dream is that we feel like we're split in two, going two or more directions when there is only one body, mind, and spirit. What we see may not be "real." When we realize and believe there's only one Spirit, one energy from which all things come, we can be at peace.

You may feel like you need help being put back together, much like Humpty Dumpty who had a great fall. If so, ask for what you need. Asking for help when you can't do it all by yourself is a sign of empowerment rather than weakness.

Tragedy, illness, and accidents often seem to bring out the best in humans. In these situations acting spontaneously in the moment with compassion seems so natural. No one is thinking about what to do next or how much money will be earned for helping someone.

All we see is a person in distress. All we think about is how we can help, or perhaps we don't think at all. We just do whatever it feels like we need to do next. We may send thoughts for healing, prayers, food, clothing, free housing, or financial donations. Perhaps we offer physical or emotional support on site.

Whatever it is, we recognized something in these people that was the same as we recognized in ourselves. It may have been our heart connecting with theirs. We may have felt a deep, loving spiritual bond with them. Most likely it is difficult to put that awareness into words. It is more of a feeling and a knowing that doesn't translate well into language.

If you've ever experienced a severe illness or accident, it may have been life changing. People who have gone through this, as I have, usually never look at themselves or others in the same way again. While the experience is frequently painful, traumatic, physically confining, and/or mentally or emotionally upsetting, ultimately it often leads to a new spiritual awareness and gratitude.

It is more of a **feeling** *and a knowing that doesn't translate well into language.*

At some point we sense we are so much more than a body and a mind. We start believing that a part of us continues and extends beyond us even after the body and mind are gone. That part is beingness or the essence of love or oneness.

Knowing and believing that this beingness or consciousness can never be lost is reassuring. It can help take away the fear of death. With this new awareness, what is it that dies? Is it you? No, it's only the body changing form. Your true essence is eternal and changeless. You are still part of the consciousness that is, the universal consciousness that everyone and everything shares.

Assisting people in the "dying" process is one of the things I do. Usually by the time a family member contacts me, the loved one is very near "death" and in a coma. By then the doctors have done all they can do to help. This person has already lived beyond what the doctors have estimated.

When I arrive, members of the family and, sometimes, friends, are gathered together, grieving and feeling helpless to do anything more. They are hoping I can facilitate a peaceful release for their loved one.

I encourage the family and friends to release any emotions or thoughts that may be keeping the person in the physical dimension, if they haven't already done so. Also, the lingering "dying" often have a fear of dying or feel they have unfinished work or relationships to heal. Then I invite Spirit, the angels and the guides, or other beings, according to the belief system

We and all of our relations are **interconnected** *as one family.*

of the family, to assist us in releasing the energy that's holding the person in the body.

After doing one or two energy techniques, I show the family how they can help after I'm gone. Usually I get a call the next day, letting me know that the individual passed on peacefully within a few hours after I left, and expressing their gratitude.

Celebrating the time of release from the body is a wonderful way of honoring someone's passing into another dimension. Since we celebrate arrival into physical form, why not celebrate our departure also?

What is the worst that can happen if you change, make an error, or use your inner power? When you no longer fear death of the body and can accept the oneness of all, you can more easily gather up the courage to release lesser fears. Without fear, you can do whatever you desire, be at peace, and experience joy. You'll freely extend love to yourself and those around you.

The essence of love is what we feel when we reach out to people, when we nurture ourselves and others, and when we are at peace with who we are. Awareness of ourselves as spiritual beings increases. Just as human beings are created by one father and mother, we realize everyone is created by the same consciousness and the same spiritual mother and father. In both cases, we and all of our relations are interconnected as one family.

Empowerment Guide

- The ego sees us as separate from everyone and everything, including Spirit.

- The ego has no power except what we choose to give it.

- Cease believing that everything you see and hear around you is truth.

- Asking for help when you really need it is empowering.

- Look at others as manifestations of Spirit, the oneness of All That Is.

- Seeing through the eyes of very young children is liberating.

- Find the truth of oneness deep within yourself.

- Choose to perceive in a way that helps you feel freer and more empowered.

- Let go of thoughts of separation, most of what you've learned about yourself and the world, and what you've thought was true.

- Without fear, including the fear of death, and a sense of separation, we can do whatever we desire, be at peace, and experience joy.

- Live your life as though Spirit lived with you in all physical forms daily.

- Our true essence is eternal and changeless.

Action Guide

Affirmations:

I acknowledge (or bless) the presence of Spirit (or oneness) in you. (Repeat this for each person you meet or communicate with during the day.)

I embrace the oneness of all people and All That Is.

Energy Technique:

Prayer is an energy form that works. All prayers are answered, can be used for yourself and others, and are also effective at a distance. Consider using them to ask for guidance, to see differently, or to find peace within yourself. If you are used to praying from the heart, then continue with what you've been doing. Use it often and see how helpful and freeing it can be. Ultimately, prayer is direct communication with higher consciousness with an emphasis on listening.

Place one or both of your hands over your heart, hold them together in prayer position, or use any other position that is comfortable for you. Ask for help in feeling love for yourself and all others. Ask to be shown how to reclaim your power from the ego and find your inner truth. You can do this in a prayer form you are familiar with or use a conversational tone as you would with a good friend, e.g. "I could use some help here. I'm really tired of the way my life is going, and I don't know what to do about it. I'm ready to listen."

Inner Connecting: Tiger Unity

Get in a comfortable position in a quiet place and close your eyes. Place one or two hands at your heart and relax your breathing. In this inner-connecting activity, focus on love, joy, peace, or healing energy. Take a moment to choose the one that feels right for you in this moment. You'll use this energy for yourself and others during this quiet, focused time.

Begin feeling this warm, soothing energy slowly filling your body, beginning with your toes, your feet, and then your legs. Continue feeling this wonderful energy spreading up into your pelvic area, your lower abdomen, upper abdomen, and your solar plexus below your heart. Next bring this energy into your heart center beneath your hands. Focus your entire attention there, allowing the energy to completely fill your heart. When that feels complete, move your attention to your throat, neck, shoulders, arms, your third eye at the center of your brow, and the top of your head.

Now return your focus to your heart center. Begin extending that energy out to those dearest to you: your spouse or partner, children, parents, grandparents, the rest of your family, your neighbors, any people with you now, the people at church and at work, and those who serve you: a massage therapist, holistic practitioners, an auto mechanic, accountant, hairdresser, medical professionals, teachers, mentors, cooks and food servers, office staff, and any others that help you.

If at any point you feel the vibration of the energy you've chosen to work with is slowing or losing power, return to your heart center and focus on increasing the energy. Then go back to extending this energy to others.

Let this energy flow to those you serve through your work, through volunteering, teaching at school or church, or helping the elderly, the disabled, and those who are ill. Spread this energy to those of other faiths, races, and cultures.

Continue sending this energy to any specific people or situations that are personally challenging to you. Perhaps it's a difficult boss, a recent loss, or financial distress. Again, if you feel the energy slowing or it feels difficult, return to your heart center as before and rebuild the energy before continuing.

Now let your attention and energy expand to include the unknown: unknown universes, unknown possibilities, people you have yet to meet, the great void, the nothingness, and the "everythingness," the All That Is. Since it's all unknown, just allow it to be, surrounding it in love, joy, peace, and healing energy.

Notice how you feel. Remember this feeling, this place of beingness. Extend this energy to people and events you interact with in your daily living.

Now smile. Take three deep breaths and open your eyes when you are ready.

You can choose to share your experience and feelings with someone nearby or someone dear to you. You can journal about it, adding any insights you may have gotten. You can let this experience go immediately, returning to this meditation as often as you like. Choose what feels best to you.

Doing inner connecting can be a useful tool for shifting your perception of the world around you. After you've done this several times, you can use a shorter version that works for you. Here's an example.

Fill your body, beingness, and space around you with the energy or emotion you've chosen to work with. Send the chosen energy out to those closest to you and then to those you do not know as well. Continue by surrounding the more challenging people and situations in your life with this vibrational frequency. Move your attention and energy to the unknown. Return to your heart center. Remember this feeling and extend it to people and events in your daily living. Smile, take three deep breaths, and open your eyes.

Namaste. I honor the God within you.

Essential Oils:

Frankincense, Canadian Red Cedar, and Western Red Cedar

- See the end of Chapter Four to review possible benefits and applications for Frankincense.
- The Red Cedar oils listed above enhance the potential for spiritual communication, awareness, and meditation. Apply them to the bottom of your feet, directly on an area of concern, or diffuse into the air.

More Steps to Tiger Unity

- Look at your beliefs. Let go of those that are not congruent with the truth of who you are. Keep those that help you see and feel the oneness of all things.

- Listen to beautiful, soothing, uplifting music that helps you relax, get quiet, and smile.

- Read and listen to inspirational stories from books, movies, and television.

- Observe ego-based thoughts, words, and emotions that take you away from peace, love, and joy. Choose thoughts and words that feel good to you.

- Look for the inner truth and beauty in each person you meet throughout the day.

- Offer a sincere compliment about a special quality or service you appreciate in the people you communicate with during the day.

- Feel a sense of oneness and an appreciation for everyone and everything around you.

Healing Guide

Since we know life in bodies is temporary, let's honor, respect, and love others, as well as ourselves, as if all were welcome guests in our homes. How would it change your experience here on earth if you knew Spirit, All That Is, lives with you in physical form every day? If you believed that was really true, what would you say, think, and do differently? Connecting with pure consciousness is how you'll discover peace, joy, and love.

Awaken your
heart's song and
dance
with joy.

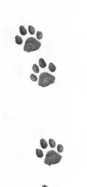

CHAPTER EIGHT

The **Tiger's** HeartSong

Healing from the Heart

AWAKEN YOUR HEART'S SONG and dance with joy. True healing comes from your heart. When you connect with the energy and wisdom of your heart, the tiger within, you also connect with the oneness that joins all people. Healing from your heart is the eighth path.

The heart, the center of love, is a faithful guide. Too often, however, we forget to be quiet and access our heart-knowing. When we do remember, we frequently don't trust it and don't follow it.

When we don't connect with our heart's wisdom, we lose the joy, the love, and the peace in our lives. We lose our sense of empowerment, our belief that we have the power to make a difference in our lives.

As a little girl, I witnessed this loss of empowerment as it manifested in both my maternal grandmother and my mother.

The heart, the center of love, is a faithful **guide.**

Joy's Family Story

My grandmother graduated from the eighth grade, considered quite an accomplishment for that time in history more than one hundred years ago. With this credential, Grandma Amelia started teaching school long before it was common for women to work outside the home. She agreed to teach in a school where the students spoke only German. Since Grandma didn't speak any German, it was definitely more of a challenge than she had anticipated. She stopped teaching after one term.

My grandparents got married just after the turn of the last century. My grandfather loaded up a Conestoga wagon the day after their wedding. He took Grandma to western South Dakota where "there was nothing but rattlesnakes," according to Grandma. Occasionally they saw another man, but usually it was just the two of them working and trying to subsist on fairly barren land.

They lived in the wagon four to five months. Then Grandpa heard how cold the winters could be there, especially without shelter. He was also concerned because his first child was due in three to four months, and there was no doctor anywhere nearby. So they returned to civilization where they'd be warmer and have access to a doctor.

Grandma Amelia absolutely hated homesteading, without any contact with women and without any of the conveniences she had enjoyed before her marriage. She had led a fairly pampered, sheltered life before her marriage, enjoying such niceties as having a dressmaker make her clothing.

Now Grandma began caring for a household, a husband and children, and learning how to make do with very little money. They raised thirteen children plus cattle, chickens, pigs, and crops. At times my grandparents were caregivers for several of their fifty-three grandchildren, including me.

Grandpa ruled over the family through fear, a strong hand, a razor strop, a switch, and anything else nearby, including his fists. Grandma was afraid of him and tried to keep the children out of his way. Everyone learned it was best to avoid my grandfather's wrath whenever possible.

As an adult, one of my uncles asked Grandma why she married someone who was even mean to the horses. She replied, "I never saw that side of him then." Apparently he was very capable of being on his best behavior when it served his purposes.

Once when my grandma was in a nursing home, Grandpa was looking at their wedding picture. He said, according to my aunt, "No one thought I could get that cute little Catholic girl." He had set out to take control and prove them wrong.

Grandpa was in charge of everything. He told Grandma she could go to church. However, they lived far away from her church, and he refused to take her. He forbade my grandma from talking about her beliefs or expressing her thoughts. In their conversations with other people, Grandma couldn't get a word in edgewise.

In later years he allowed her to attend the Ladies' Aid Society once a month. When Grandpa found a church *he* wanted to go to, Grandma was encouraged to go with him.

Grandma was a petite woman with a big, generous heart. She very capably managed, cared for, fed, clothed, and guided her large family. Yet, she did not feel free to do what she wanted to do or to speak her truth. Because Grandma didn't feel her desires made any difference and feared retribution, she did what my grandfather told her to do. This is a classic example of loss of empowerment.

My mother was the youngest girl in the family. She heard her older brothers and sisters talking about leaving home just as soon as they could figure out how to do it. Mom watched as some of her brothers and one sister left home to join the military; others left to get a job to escape from my grandfather's heavy hand and make it on their own.

Mom got out of her parents' house by marrying my father, a neighboring farm boy, when she was sixteen. I was born during their first year of marriage. We lived with my paternal grandparents for a short time. Grandma Goldie was every bit as much of a tyrant as my maternal grandpa was. She had eight children. She ruled harshly over her five sons and three daughters and her alcoholic husband, Grandpa Frank.

Grandma Goldie's heart was angry and bitter. She spewed venom at all who came close to her. Although she wielded "power" over others, she wasn't connecting with and using her true power. Grandma Goldie wasn't happy, peaceful, or compassionate.

Mom finally couldn't endure the situation any longer. She took me with her and left my dad and his parents' house. Mom struggled to find work, going from one type of unskilled labor to another throughout her life. When she felt threatened in some way, unhappy with someone, or fearful, she shouted a lot and lashed out at me or anyone else who had provoked her anger, sometimes throwing dishes or anything else nearby. Mom expressed her anger much as her father did.

My mother always seemed to be looking for someone else or something outside herself to make her happy. She was usually living with a man and married most of them. Over time I lost count of the number of stepfathers I had. What I saw growing up was that my mom always chose a man with similar characteristics as the last one she had lived with (except for my father). She rebounded from one to another, never satisfied with any of them for long.

Joy's Story
Childhood Challenges

I learned at a very early age to take care of myself. I learned I was very uncomfortable being around people with loud, argumentative, demanding voices, and also physically and emotionally abusive people. I learned I didn't like feeling abandoned. As a child coming out of this tradition, I was determined not to follow in the footsteps of my mom and grandma.

As a young child, I was physically and sexually abused. The sexual abuse ended when Mom left one of my stepfathers. The belt lashings stopped when I became strong enough to take the belt away from my mother at about age ten. Looking back, I see this act as another early example of beginning to claim and use my power.

All of these experiences caused me to cringe, retreat into myself, read the Bible, sit quietly in secluded trees, and turn to a power within and beyond myself. I heard a message from deep inside my heart that said, "There's more to life than you've experienced so far." I wanted to believe that was true and began looking for it. Now I see these periods of quiet contemplation as the beginning of my search for the tiger, the power within.

When I was thirteen, we were running from the law. My mom's boyfriend was being hunted down. We stayed with one of his relatives for a short time in the country. I was attending a small rural school. One day Mom said, "Come on. We're leaving." These words were all too familiar. They always meant one of two things. Either I was going to be abandoned once again, or I'd be running away with Mom from some "intolerable" situation to some unknown place.

"There's more to **life** *than you've experienced so far."*

This time I said, "No. I don't want to go with you."

Mom said, "What will you do?"

I responded, "My teacher said I could live with her if I needed a place to stay."

Mom talked to my teacher, who agreed to take me in. I never lived with my mom again. My father already had more children living with him from another marriage than he could comfortably support. He thought I would have more opportunities in foster care.

I was placed in foster care with my teacher's family and felt blessed to have two wonderful sets of foster parents and my "sisters" until high school graduation. I witnessed and experienced love, trust, happiness, having enough, and a belief in dreams with these very special people.

More of Mom's Story

Mom continued her pattern of unsuccessful relationships, frequent job changes, running away from difficult situations, and searching for love the rest of her life. She was always looking for a happier life and never found it. Her last husband took her life and then his own. Mom was forty-three and had not learned she had the power to change her life and find true happiness.

My mother never learned how to look inside herself and follow her heart. She didn't believe she deserved any more than she had. Mom never asked herself what kind of life she wanted, believed she could have it, or took steps to create it. She felt totally powerless to make a difference in her life, just like her mother.

Joy's Story
Adulthood Loss of Joy

Meanwhile, I married, had children, graduated from college, and led a very "respectable" life. I was a "successful" career woman, working in education as Grandma Amelia once did, and trying to balance family, finances, work, and play.

Since I was determined not to be like my mother (no matter what) and converted to Catholicism (my husband's religion), I was committed to making my marriage work even though my husband was emotionally abusive to me and others closest to him. He seemed to have a need to be in control and to put others down to make himself feel better.

Due to my strong desire never to fall victim to the patterns of my mother, I swung the other way with the pendulum. Instead of knowing what I wanted and believing I could have it, I tried to avoid what I didn't want just as Grandma Amelia and Mom did. Specifically... I wanted to avoid divorce.

As the years went by, I became unhappier with my relationship, but still I was reluctant to give up on it. Eventually, my husband left the state with a much younger woman. Thus our marriage ended after nearly thirty years.

I truly felt grateful and free. My relationship with my husband had been very difficult for years. However, because of my limiting belief about staying married for life, I chose not to follow what my heart was telling me.

Reflecting on this experience, I see that I made some of the same choices Grandma Amelia did. I realize now if I had listened to my inner guidance instead of resisting it, I would have left my marriage years earlier and used my power to make the choices that would have brought me joy and peace much sooner.

I truly felt **grateful** *and free.*

Now I was free but physically ill. The many years of stressful living and ignoring my heart's wisdom had weakened my immune system. This, in turn, made me very susceptible to the pesticide poisoning which occurred just months after my divorce.

Do I blame anyone for what happened? No. Am I looking for sympathy or empathy? Definitely not. The experiences I've had all shape who I am today. My past has brought me to a place of knowing the truth of who I am and feeling a desire to speak my truth.

I share this vignette from my life story as another example of how we give our power away or fail to use it. Perhaps you identify with one of these women or one of my grandfathers. Are you still "stuck" in a victim role or in a controlling role? Or have you moved beyond the fear, anger, and hurt to a place of healing from your heart?

As long as you continue to act like a victim, repeating the pattern you're in, and feeling helpless to change the situation, you're blocking your power. Become aware of what's happening. See how you feel about it, learn from it, let go of the past, and move on. You don't need to stay stuck in an energy-draining or potentially unsafe set of circumstances.

We always have choices, no matter how difficult or impossible it may seem. Another way out of a situation is always available if you believe it, are open to it, and ask for help. Neither Grandma Amelia nor my mom believed it and suffered as a result.

You can always break out of family patterns, just as I did. It doesn't matter whether it is related to abuse, addictions, poverty, health, education, or something else. In my case, I didn't learn to claim and use my power overnight. If you asked me when I started listening to and following my heart, I would have to say, "It has been a process of listening, knowing, resisting, and following in different degrees over time."

Since I sensed and trusted life could be more than my current experience of it, I was open to something other than what I had manifested in my life so far. Some of my life experiences stand out as small but significant steps on my journey to discovering and using my power. Quiet contemplation as a young child set the tone and practice of searching inside.

Having the courage to take the belt away from my mother at age ten was significant and gave me a glimpse of how my choices could bring about a desired outcome. Telling my mother at age thirteen that I didn't want to go with her was a turning point in my life. This time I was listening and following my heart. I knew continuing to run and hide didn't feel good to me. I had the courage to stand up to my mother once again, even though it meant living with and trusting people I had just met. Somehow I knew I would be safe and well cared for.

During my long marriage, I listened and followed in some ways and not in others. Another major shift in discovering my power occurred when my marriage ended. Now I was able to see that the thing I had resisted the most was actually a path to freedom and empowerment. In subsequent relationships, I have practiced my right to choose, making choices from a place of empowerment, breaking the patterns followed by my mom and Grandma Amelia.

With the onset of the environmental illness and related health conditions, I began listening and following more consistently. I realized I was the only one interested in finding answers to this health dilemma. I also knew that I didn't have a clue what to do even though I had always considered myself a fairly self-sufficient person. I focused on listening to my heart more, strengthening my intuition, and following the subtle guidance that eventually led me to significant improvement in my health and a sense of greater empowerment.

As I look back, I realize I could have made different choices along the way. Yet who can say that one choice was right and another was wrong? I followed my guidance as well as I could for where I was on my path. That's all anyone can do. If you're not happy, you can always choose again.

The real commitment is to listen to your heart all the time. This can happen much easier and quicker than you think is possible. Let go of judgment, believe in yourself, and turn to the tiger within.

The real commitment is to listen to your heart all the time.

The heart is not just a metaphor for love, inner guidance, and emotional expression. Physically, in addition to its circulatory function, the heart guides us and controls other bodily functions. Scientists used to tell us that the brain controlled the body. Now we know that the heart actually controls much of the brain. The heart also retains memories, likes, and dislikes, including food preferences, choice of vocabulary, and much more.

We can learn a lot from the heart by listening to it on different levels. Physically you may feel pain or tightness. You may check your pulse, blood pressure, or cholesterol on a regular basis. You may go to a doctor to have a battery of tests done.

Mentally you may wonder what's going on. Why is this happening now? To help you at this level, review what was happening prior to noticing the symptoms. Is it an ongoing situation? These questions and similar ones will start giving you clues about your heart's message.

What do other people say to you or in your presence? All of these words will give you clues about what's happening to your heart.

Listen to the words you use when talking about yourself, your life, and your heart. Here are some familiar phrases: broken heart, heavy heart, heartaches, stabbed in the heart, lonely heart, heart cries out, poured out my heart, hard-hearted, and heart attack. What's hurting your heart? Who or what is attacking it?

We also have many expressions about happy, loving hearts: touched my heart, tugged at my heartstrings, my heart goes out to you, my heart sings, my heart is jumping for joy, and kind-hearted. Do any of these resonate with you? What do they relate to?

What can you do to shift and lighten the energy around your heart? What lifestyle changes you can make to slow your pace, relieve stress, and allow more time for rest and relaxation? Consider changes you can make in your diet, job, habits, or living situation.

The heart is the seat of many emotions: feeling unloved, abandoned, insecure, unappreciated, disconnected from your emotions, and having difficulty expressing your emotions, to name just a few. The heart and how you talk about it give you valuable information about yourself.

Can you identify experiences prior to your heart symptoms that evoked any of these emotions? The emotional energy from past experiences can get "stuck" in your heart, causing the energy eventually to block up. You can use some of the techniques at the end of this chapter to help release these emotions. However, it can also be very beneficial to get professional help.

Jerry's Story

For example, one day as I started working with Jerry to repattern and clear an allergy, I noticed the energy at both the heart chakra and the sacral area was very congested and out of balance. After sharing this with Jerry, he said, "My best friend died. I just came back from attending his funeral out of state."

The energy pattern I felt is very typical for clients who have experienced a recent loss. The sacral chakra is, in part, about relationships. The heart, in Jerry's case, was about feeling abandoned. I released, cleared, and balanced the energy in these chakras. After I finished, Jerry said, "I feel lighter, happier, and more energized."

Emotions play a huge role in the development of disease in the body. Breast cancer and lung problems also are related to the same emotions as the heart.

Lacy's Story

Lacy, another client, asked me to help her release "stuck" emotional energy. The energy around and above her physical heart felt very congested and dense. Lacy has difficulty sharing on an emotional level. She seems to think it's a sign of weakness to feel or talk about sensitive emotions and lacks clarity about what emotions she's feeling. I focused on repairing Lacy's emotional heart. After this session she said, "I feel lighter and freer."

When we feel disconnected or out of touch with our feelings, abandoned, or unloved, it's often an indication of feeling disconnected from Spirit, from the divine essence of love and peace.

Unconditional love is something we all yearn for and seldom experience. Unconditional love accepts others and allows them to be just as they are. It means not judging and comparing or trying to change someone. Unconditional love means feeling compassion for all people. It means honoring where each person is in her life journey. It means extending love no matter what someone has done or not done.

Unconditional love doesn't mean we condone or support someone's behavior or agree with it. It doesn't mean we will want to be best friends with everyone. We don't need to open our home to all the homeless or "down on their luck" people. However, we might choose to do volunteer work at a local shelter or raise funds to help those in need.

How would your life be different if you had someone that you could share anything with and still feel loved and supported? Can you be that kind of person for someone else?

Imagine how the world would change if you, and everyone else, felt loved for who you are, without conditions, instead of for what you do. Imagine how you'd feel if you knew you didn't need to be smarter, nicer looking, more creative, more hard-working, neater, more religious, or more spiritual to be loved.

When we feel love for ourselves, others, and All That Is, our very presence is healing. This is referred to as healing presence. When we emit that energy, others feel it and are drawn to us.

Strangers may come up to you and start a conversation. People may start pouring out their story to you. If you spend time with someone who is ill or discouraged, he may begin feeling better because your energy has helped raise his energetic vibration.

Listening without judgment, sitting with someone in silence, holding someone's hand, or speaking truth from deep in your heart are all very healing when we come from a place of being fully present in love.

Offering sincere, loving words describing what you appreciate or have observed about another person is very healing and energizing. For example:

- Your smile always lights up the room.

- You have such a wonderful gift for words. You always seem to know just the right thing to say to help someone else feel better.

- I feel such a deep sense of peace when I'm with you.

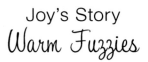

Joy's Story
Warm Fuzzies

I once taught a class on healing words to a group of about fifteen women. One of the activities I asked them to do was to write one or two positive comments about each woman in the room. Not all the women knew everyone well. In those cases, I suggested they simply focus quietly on the woman and write something from their heart to her heart. The women gave their comments or "warm fuzzies" to each other and took them home to read.

The next time we got together, the women were still talking about how great they felt reading their warm fuzzies. One woman said, "I decided to wait awhile before reading mine. Then one day when I was feeling a little down, I looked at them. I can't describe how wonderful I felt reading them. Now I've been reading them every day and smiling. I didn't know other people would say such nice things about me."

How would you feel if someone, even an anonymous someone, gave you a warm fuzzy? How would you feel if you got one a week or even one a day?

Imagine how would you feel if you gave a warm fuzzy a day to someone without identifying yourself. How do you think the other person would feel?

I encourage you to give sincere heartfelt compliments to people you know—family, friends, and coworkers—as well as to those you don't know well. What if it caught on and other people started giving them out daily? How would that change the way people feel about themselves and those they work and play with?

Passion
is your heart's desire.

Think about what brings you true joy. Do you know what "lights your fire" and makes you feel like dancing and singing in the wind?

What is *your* passion? Can you feel a shift in your energy when you're speaking about your passion or following it? Others can.

Passion is your heart's desire. It comes from deep inside, from connecting with your inner self. Passion is what excites you and makes you feel good all over. It's also what you want to spend more time doing.

You can tell when others are passionate about something. You can sense their enthusiasm, feel the energy with which they speak, and see a sparkle in their eyes. It's as though their whole being comes more alive.

If you still aren't sure what your passion is, start paying attention to your feelings. What feels good and what doesn't? When you pay close attention to your feelings and use them as a guide for finding your passion, you become more powerful and feel more connected to All That Is. Ask a friend or family member to help you identify your passion if you feel a need for more help.

When you find your passion, start making time to pursue it. At first you may feel you don't have the time to do anything with it. Begin with whatever amount of time you can work into your schedule, even if it's just a few minutes a day.

You'll have more energy and enthusiasm *for life.*

Notice how you feel when you start taking steps toward following your passion. The more you do, the more excited you'll become. As the excitement builds, you'll find you're spending more time focusing on your passion. You'll begin feeling different about yourself. You'll have more energy and enthusiasm for life.

Creating what you desire begins with taking action to change how you feel about yourself and your life. Focus on adding more fun and passion in your life and experience the joy of being.

Have you ever felt your heart ached, you were stabbed in the back or your heart was heavy? Have you suffered from loss or grief perhaps following death, divorce, or disaster? If so, you may have closed off your heart to protect yourself from further emotional pain. When you do that, your heart, lungs, and breasts suffer an energetic loss.

Then energy in the aura, as well as in the physical body, becomes denser and more congested. This, in turn, slows down the flow of energy throughout your body resulting in illness, reduced connection with others, and possibly death. Often when a beloved spouse dies, the surviving spouse dies of a "broken heart" within a few days to a year later.

If you close off or shut down your emotional heart, you may have a heart attack or turn into someone we describe as "hard-hearted" or a lonely heart. You may protest and say, "But it hurts too much. I don't want to be hurt again." If you keep guarding your heart, you cannot feel joy, passion, or peace in your life.

Recently more clients are coming to me with broken hearts and other energetic heart issues. Sometimes their complaints relate to areas adjacent to the heart such as lungs, pancreas, or ribs. Some ask for help releasing blockages that are keeping them from moving forward with what they really want to do. In other cases, as I'm doing an assessment, I find that the energy around the heart is not flowing well.

A large percentage of my clients have energetic heart issues. However, most are not aware of this. They may have high blood pressure but have not been diagnosed with any heart condition.

I love working with people at this stage because we're releasing congested energy at the heart before serious physical symptoms appear. The client and I work together to heal the energetic heart. This can help prevent more severe problems from arising. This work also helps heal the heart on all levels. This allows clients to open their hearts more to them-selves and others and move through some emotional blockages.

More of Paula's Story

Paula recently contracted a virus that settled in her lungs. She is the client with cystic fibrosis whom you met earlier. For her, this can be a life-threatening situation. Paula was working with her doctor, who said, "If it doesn't get better soon, we'll have to put you back on anti-biotics intravenously."

Since the energy that flows through the lungs and ribs is affected by the heart chakra, I always clear any energy congestion in these areas first. After I finished releasing congested energy around Paula's lungs, I discovered the energy at her heart center was very dense and stuck, much like a rock. Paula said, "It feels very heavy there."

Using my intuition, I worked in the energy field and released some dense, heavy energy about thirty inches above her body. Paula said, "What was that? I felt something leave."

Paula followed my voice guidance, breathing and visualizing as I worked to clear away some of the "stuck" energy around the heart. Her heart chakra had several energetic breaks in it also. I repaired them and adjusted the chakra energy so it stopped wobbling and started spinning smoothly and evenly.

Next I directed a focused, aligned yellow crystal energy coming from my hands and reached down to a deep cellular level with it. This aligned and balanced the heart energy. (This crystal energy shifts the chaotic energy from beliefs, habits, emotions, thoughts, stress, and more. It also raises the energetic vibration and brings the heart energy into resonance with the rest of the body.)

Paula held some Biogenesis™ healing tools that have proven to be so helpful to her. Meanwhile I repaired the energetic grid around her heart through all of the levels of the energy field: physical, emotional, mental, and spiritual. It seems a little like repairing very fine mesh, except I'm working multidimensionally.

When we finished this session, Paula said, "I feel so much better. I can breathe easier, and the heaviness is gone. Two days later Paula called to report. "Congratulations! I don't need the antibiotics. Good job!"

I replied, "Congratulations to you! You're the one who really did the healing work."

We can learn to listen to the wisdom of the heart. Sometimes, even when we desire it with our minds, we still feel something is blocking our ability to fully open our hearts. If this is happening to you, you can follow some of the suggestions at the end of this chapter or consult with a professional trained to help you release emotional or energetic blockages relating to your heart.

Empowerment Guide

- Speaking from our heart is healing.
- Listen to your heart. Pay attention to the words you and others use in talking about the heart.
- Believe that you have the power to make a difference in your life.
- To discover your passion, connect with your feelings.
- Following our passion will create energy and enthusiasm for life.
- True healing comes from the heart, from that place deep inside us.

Action Guide

Affirmations:

I make choices from a place of quiet knowing.
I embrace love and truth in each moment.
My heart is filled with joy.

Energy Technique:

Using either one or two hands, gently clear the energy field above the heart. Start with your hand(s) near the heart. Then move your hand(s) out and away from your heart into the energy field beyond your body and release the energy. Visualizing what it would feel like to move your hands from the center of a cloud to the edge and beyond may be helpful. Do this for 20-30 seconds or more.

Next hold your hands over your heart chakra for one to three minutes while breathing gently and deeply. Send warm, loving, healing energy to your heart while holding your hands in place.

Inner Connecting: Tiger Heart

Sit in a quiet place in a comfortable position. Begin relaxing your body by focusing on your breathing—in and out, in and out. With each exhale, blow out worry, stress, and tension. With each inhale, breathe in peace, love, and joy.

Feel your body relaxing...relaxing...relaxing. Your mind is getting quieter and quieter. Now you're beginning to become more aware of your body: warmth, tingling, respiration, and heartbeat. Notice what you're feeling.

Turn your attention to your heart. What are you noticing in and around the physical heart? Whatever it is, just allow it to be. With each breath, allow anything from the physical body that is ready to release, to release gently and easily.

Begin letting your attention go deeper into your emotional heart. What are you feeling: sensations...emotions... or something else? If there's anything you're ready to release emotionally, allow it to release.

Is one emotion stronger than the others? Are you getting a sense of what that is about? Does your emotional heart have a message for you? It may come in the form of a physical sensation, a memory flashing into your awareness, words, a knowing, or an emotional response such as tears or a feeling of peace.

Now let's go deeper and begin focusing on your mental heart. What thoughts or words are coming to you? Allow whatever comes up just to be. Be open to releasing whatever is ready to be released.

Let's go deeper yet into the spiritual heart, that place of being. What do you notice there? Are you getting a sense of what's happening in this place? Be willing to let go of whatever is willing to be released. Listen carefully for a message of healing from that place of inner knowing...deep in your heart.

Where is your inner tiger? Can you see it or feel it? If you need help getting clarity about what's in the spiritual heart, ask your tiger to help. Take some time getting to know and trust your tiger.

Now gradually begin shifting your attention back through the layers of your heart from the spiritual to the mental...then to the emotional heart...and the physical heart.

You will remember your messages and your guidance. If you aren't aware of any messages, ask for more clarity. A message may come to you later.

Gently move your hands to your heart and let them rest there for a moment. Feel the love and peace in your heart building in power and intensity. Feel your heart opening wider and wider and deeper and deeper. Notice how that feels. Feel your heart healing at all levels. Feel how deeply connected you are to All That Is.

Know that it's safe to open your heart. Know that it's safe to keep it open. Know that you'll heal your heart by opening it and keeping it open.

Now bring your attention back to your physical body...to your breathing...and to the floor or ground beneath you. Wiggle your fingers and toes. Open your eyes when you're ready.

Essential Oils:

Lavender and Ylang Ylang

- Lavender has cardio-tonic, regenerative, anti-inflammatory, and anticoagulant properties. It may help with tachycardia and high blood pressure. Apply directly to your feet and heart areas and diffuse into the air.

- Ylang Ylang may reduce arterial hypertension, palpitations, tachycardia, and blood pressure. Regular use may balance heart function and release emotional energy congestion.

More Steps to the Tiger's Heart

- Follow your heart-knowing.

- Focus on feeling love for All That Is, for all people, for the earth, and for yourself.

- Find special ways of showing the love you feel for others: spouse, children, coworkers, teachers, friends, service providers, homeless, handicapped, abandoned animals, strangers, and more. A smile, a helping hand, quality time, or a "warm fuzzy" will usually convey the message better than money or a superficial compliment ever could.

- Choose a book that gives you insight, inspiration, comfort, or guidance. What guidance or clarity are you seeking? Open the book to any page and read the section that catches your attention. You may be amazed at how well that will address your question.

Healing Guide

Release your fears and let go of resistance to life experiences to increase your energy. The energy to, through, and from your heart will then flow more freely and easily. This will also help you heal your heart. Through opening your heart, you can be and flow with what is, love more fully, and experience the oneness, the All That Is. You can only feel love when you open your heart and keep it open.

By walking through life
one step at a time and
getting to know the

truth

of who you are, you'll find
that life is about being

fully present

with what is.

CHAPTER NINE

The Zen
Tiger
Being and Flowing

FROM A PLACE OF HEART-KNOWING, being and flowing is a natural process on the journey of healing and empowerment and is the ninth path. Fear, doubt, failure, and excuses for not following our heart's desires and guidance do not exist as reasons for not pursuing our dreams. We'll simply go around any temporary roadblocks.

With this awareness, we'll perceive any challenges we encounter along the way as opportunities to be creative and listen more closely to our guidance. The ninth path is being fully in the moment and coming from presence. From this place we'll discover and use our power.

Joy's Dream

This recent dream speaks to a sense of empowerment.

I am outdoors with one hundred or more people. Whenever I feel like doing something, it just happens. I am very confident. Everything is easy and flows well.

I am aware others are watching me, enjoying the ease, grace, and flow they are witnessing. I entertain people effort-

lessly, with no thought. I can fly easily, maneuvering in any direction and doing whatever I choose with no challenges or errors.

A man is nearby being supportive and watching. He can do some of the same things I am doing. It seems that the other people don't believe they can.

Feeling healed and empowered requires moving beyond fear and negativity. What do you want your life to be like? See it, believe it, release it, and do it. Since you're already healed spiritually and are empowered by your state of beingness, it's really about letting go of everything that isn't love and truth.

Stacy's Story

Stacy's adult life exemplifies being and flowing with what is. If she wants her life to look a little different, she takes steps to change it rather than complaining about it. If one part of her life is cut off, she pursues another. She did not blame others for any of her life experiences.

Stacy's passion for dancing led her to an opportunity to dance for money in the clubs before age nineteen. Stacy described herself in her younger years as tall, smart, and pretty with a good figure but not as striking as many of the other dancers. She watched other dancers to discover the difference between those who were getting more tip money and those who were getting less.

In her first month of dancing for pay, Stacy noted that an ugly dancer made $400 in tips while she took in just $50. Obviously it had very little to do with physical appearance. Stacy learned that if she did table dancing, dancing at the tables as the ugly girl did, she made a lot more money.

According to Stacy, exotic dancers don't have to be able to dance. The primary criterion is the size of the boobs. "Some of the girls had boobs bigger than their heads, but they couldn't dance. They were all boobs and no brains (although some *were* really smart). The other two categories of dancers were magazine stars (which I wasn't) and porn stars (which I wasn't willing to do)." She said, "I didn't fit into any of the categories, so I created a new one: spectacular, artful dancing with a creative show. I was a pretty good dancer; I did it for the art."

In spite of these "handicaps," Stacy quickly became a very successful exotic dancer. Both the public and the other girls loved her dancing and her creative performances. By this time, Stacy was creating her own headliner shows and traveling a lot. Inspirations for her shows came from the songs she heard. She'd hear a song and see an entire original routine complete with props, costume, special effects, and fanfare. Stacy did fire shows, spaceship shows, and shower shows, and used other imaginative, attention-getting themes.

On one of her trips, Stacy was driving her pickup truck, as she usually did, pulling a trailer filled with her props, costumes, and equipment. After stopping at a motel for the night and not sleeping well, Stacy got back on the road., She fell asleep at the wheel, hit the median, popped off the trailer, and flipped over. Her neck was broken. It was one week after her twenty-seventh birthday.

The doctors told Stacy she would never walk again. She said, "That was okay. But no one ever told me I wouldn't be able to use my hands either. That was the really hard part. I really liked to sew."

"I have no one to blame for the accident. I just fell asleep driving. But you know what?" Stacy continued. "It's time to move on. I've got to pay attention to what's important now."

After several months in rehab and four months at home, Stacy was back in the hospital. She was diagnosed with a form of fasciitis, commonly known as a flesh-eating disease. For six months, the doctors told her she was dying. Stacy chose to live. When the doctors said, "Do this and take that," she said, "Tell me why, and I'll decide if I want to or not."

After thirteen months in the hospital and the amputation of one foot, Stacy once again returned home. "One of the first things I did was to kick my husband out of the house." Four years later, she had to have the other foot amputated.

Stacy leads a very full life. She is employed part-time, attends many special functions and activities, and is constantly learning new things.

Here's a remarkable example of Stacy's positive attitude and her ability to flow with her physical challenges. A few years ago, she received a call from the girls' soccer team coordinator. The man said they were short soccer coaches and were trying to find someone to coach her daughter's team. Stacy replied that she was in a wheelchair and wouldn't be able to help.

Then she said, "I thought about it later and decided I didn't want to use my handicap as an excuse. I was sure I could get up and down the field in my motorized wheelchair. I called the man back and told him I'd do it if they couldn't find anyone else." Shortly thereafter, Stacy became the new coach.

Stacy said laughingly, "The first thing I did was to go to the library and get a book on soccer. I read it three times. The first soccer game I ever saw was the one I coached." She said after four years of coaching, the girls continue to ask if they can be on her team.

Dancing is still a part of Stacy's life in her dreams. She says, "I dance a lot in my dreams, and I'm always in thigh-high boots so no one knows." In other dreams, Stacy's not always disabled even though the wheelchair is present. Sometimes she hops out of the chair, picks it up, and lifts it over the curb. The message in these dreams may be that Stacy believes she can do anything she desires without using her physical condition as an excuse.

Stacy agreed to share some "words of wisdom" (even though she says she doesn't feel very wise).

- Focus on what makes you happy. Life's too short to be unhappy.

- Why on earth would you wait around for someone to do for you what you can do for yourself? Strength is a core thing that says you need to take care of you.

- You can stress out about it or just go on. When someone's trying to push your buttons, don't let your buttons be pushed.

- Ask what's going on so you can make a good choice about what to do.

- You need to create what you want. You have to be able to see it to believe it. When you really want something, it seems to come to you.

As you can probably tell by now, Stacy is not a quitter. She doesn't give up when things get tough. Stacy doesn't make excuses for her life, her handicaps, or her choices. She looks for how she can accomplish something instead of complaining or whining about why she can't do it. If she had listened to other people or her ego, quite possibly she wouldn't be alive today.

Stacy appreciates synchronicities and small gifts from the universe and gives gratitude for what she has. Stacy has a passion for learning new things, for doing things well, and for following her joy. She trusts in herself and her abilities to focus, visualize, and create.

Does Stacy use her inner power? Absolutely! She is a beautiful example of empowerment, which she demonstrates through her words, actions, and life journey. She says what she thinks, does what feels right to her, and believes in herself and her ability to make wise choices. She allows and flows with what is without resistance, making adjustments as required by circumstances.

So...do you let your thoughts and your story get in your way and limit what you can create? Are you following your passion or whining and making excuses for your "stuckness"?

Being and flowing can become a way of living and seeing ourselves and the world around us. The following dream also relates to this.

Joy's Dream

I park my car and turn off the engine. The car starts rolling downhill toward a house with me still in it. I don't do anything except prepare for death since it seems imminent. I sense the brakes are useless. I am terrified, but not of death itself. What is about to happen seems inevitable. I don't call out for help. I wait for a crash or a sense of stopping. I get neither. I let go of the fear and expect a sense of release or peace. I get neither.

I am unaware of anything happening. I am not experiencing any emotion or pain or any other physical sense. I just am. I'm everything and nothing or no-thing. I've shifted from being a body with fears and limitations to a pure state of being.

One of the messages of this dream is that the way out of the maze of worldly concerns and fears is to release them and transcend the physical limitations. When we can see them from a different, more peaceful, perspective, we'll be in the flow of beingness or oneness.

Zen moments can hit us at strange times. They're the ones when everything seems to stop, and we feel totally filled with the peace and bliss of the moment. They are usually infrequent and unsought. They seem to happen whether we feel worthy or not, ready or not, looking for enlightenment or not.

Thomas' Story

This particular experience happened at a time when Thomas was unhappy with the world. He dwelled on that unhappiness with far too much intensity. He was overweight, smoked cigarettes, and was short of breath and in a lot of pain most of the time. He grudgingly forced himself to go for a walk after some urging.

This is his short story.

I trudged up the hill. It was a sunny day, but I didn't enjoy it. I got to the top of the hill—just barely. Then I stopped to catch my breath. I was hoping that I would have a fatal heart attack right there and then. No such luck. I started the trudge back home. As I rounded the corner to the next downhill leg of my walk, I heard a loud, clear, beautiful bird song. I looked up and spotted the offending bird high up in a tall tree. It was far off in the distance, but I swear it was looking right at me. Our eyes met. A great peace came over me. The moment lasted a few seconds and was gone. I finished walking home with a sense of total peace and ease.

Laurie's Story

This is one of those unforgettable, magical moments—Laurie had it when she was fourteen.

I was walking through the woods near my house on a still, overcast day. As I looked ahead, I saw this awesome sight. The sun was shining brightly through the clouds in one small glade of trees, lighting them up differently from the rest of the world. I stopped and stood there in awe. An almost magical feeling came over me as I was drawn into the center of the trees. I sat there in a state of bliss and peace basking in this special moment.

Joy's Story
Following the Trail

The following experience of being and flowing occurred one day when I felt a strong urge just to be and connect at a deep level with All That Is .

When I set out for a hike in Garden of the Gods Park in Colorado Springs recently, I knew I wanted to go to a place where I would be alone; a quiet, peaceful place without traffic noise or other people. I love people and the healing work I do, but I also love taking time just for me.

My heart is **singing!**

Now I find myself turning away from one of my favorite spots and parking in a lot I seldom use. Hmm. "Interesting," I think. "So why am I here?" I notice a trail leading up the hill and decide to follow it. Where will this take me? I don't know, but it feels right. The sun is shining warmly on my face, my hair is gently blowing in the breeze, the flow of fresh air through my nostrils and lungs is invigorating. My heart is singing! Yes, today is going to be a great day no matter where I go.

I hike wherever I choose to go, feeling as though I am being led to a special spot or on a great adventure. I come to another turning point on the path. I stop to listen deep inside to find my direction. Soon I come to a quiet secluded place—a perfect spot for reflecting and connecting with the trees, the rocks, and the hikers and bikers far below my aerie perch. Again my heart speaks. "This feels so good!"

After a little while I resume my hiking in still unfamiliar terrain—high above and apart from the world (or so it seems). I continue walking where I feel guided to go. Then as I look down, I see deer tracks and large cat tracks. They are fresh and easier to spot due to the recent, most welcome, rain.

I begin following the tracks anticipating that I might see a deer at any moment. When the tracks disappear, I continue downhill away from my car. Suddenly as I stop once again to see which way I am to go...there she is, lying on a trail to my right. Even though she jumps up quickly, she stands still a moment. Then she walks toward me until she is about fifteen feet away and stops.

Her gentle doe eyes seem so soft and loving. She is facing me, trying to catch my upwind scent. She stands there for a minute or two looking at me with those big, beautiful, brown eyes. Then she turns and walks out of view. I stay glued to my spot in stillness, listening with heightened awareness.

As I wait, she appears in front of me again walking out of the dense undergrowth. She stands on the trail in full view once more as if to say, "Oh, you're still there. I was just checking." A slight movement to her left caught my attention. It is then that I see her fawn partially concealed by the bushes. After watching me for another minute, the doe moves quietly to her left and disappears with her fawn.

I choose another path and say, "If I am to see the deer again, it will be from this trail." Several minutes later, as I am taking a careful, quiet step, I see her standing in a clearing just off the trail looking at me. I can almost hear her saying, "Oh, there you are. I've been waiting for you." She looks at me a few seconds, then turns and walks into the dense cover.

Reflecting on this experience, I realize I could have taken any path on this day; none would have been wrong. The choices I made were the right ones for me at that time. They brought me face to face with the deer. Would I have seen the deer if I had taken a different trail? I don't know. Anything is possible. I do believe my intent to see deer and my choices in the moment helped create this encounter.

In many ways my journey throughout life resembles the one I took through Garden of the Gods. It has been in large part determined by the choices I have made. Sometimes I took time to listen before acting. Other times not. My path as a healer and teacher has taken many turns and has taught me much. One thing I've learned is that it's easier to know which way to go when I take time to stop, ask quietly for guidance, and listen for the answers.

It is up to you to hear and **follow** *this guidance.*

I believe the deer crossed my path on that day to bring me a message that I feel guided to share with you. Listening quietly I heard, "There is nothing to fear. See, I do not fear you. I am only here to watch, listen, and guide you. It is up to you to hear and follow this guidance.

Whether we are venturing into new ways of being and doing, blazing a trail for others to follow, or just being makes no difference. We have the ability to see more than we can see with our eyes and know more than we can know with our minds. Just listen to that wise voice deep inside: our inner guidance."

Are you open to new opportunities and experiences, or are you trapped by the trees along the path that have grown up all around you? Is fear keeping you from exploring new trails and new ways of doing things? Perhaps it's time to really listen and face your fears as the doe in the Garden did. By walking toward me and getting to know me, she found that I was nothing to fear. By walking through life one step at a time and getting to know the truth of who you are, you'll find that life is nothing to fear.

So...do you know where *you're* going? You may be comfortable with having a plan, a road map of sorts, a general guide for your journey of healing and empowerment. Okay. So ask, "What are some ways I can get there? What do I feel drawn to do? What makes me feel good inside?" However, it's not about *where* you're going. The answer is that joy is found in letting go of attachment to the outcome, in following the path, and being peaceful in the moment—not in arriving at a destination.

Empowerment Guide

- Take time to stop, listen to, and follow your heart and your guidance.

- Choose your path in the moment from a place of knowing. All you need is enough light to see the next step.

- Remember...every path you choose is the right one for this moment.

- Release your fears to find inner peace.

- Find ways to do what you desire instead of making excuses for why you can't.

- Increase your awareness by learning to see differently and knowing more than your mind knows.

- Enjoy life and be peaceful with it no matter where it takes you.

- Let go of everything that isn't love and truth.

Action Guide

Affirmation:

I allow and flow with All That Is .

Energy Technique:

Go to a crystal shop. See which crystal(s) or stone(s) you are most attracted to. Hold your hands on or near that crystal. How does it feel to you? Are you attracted to its color, pattern, size, texture, energy, or something else? Try several. Crystals and stones historically have different energetic frequencies that can help shift your energy. Ask what the qualities are or look them up in a reference book most likely available in the same shop. Is it helpful for giving strength, protection, physical benefit, increased spiritual awareness, or something else?

Choose a crystal or stone that is small enough to easily carry with you or wear. Ask how to cleanse it. After clearing unwanted energies from it, hold it when you can easily get into a quiet, peaceful place within. Infuse that energy into the stone.

If you're feeling uneasy, challenged, afraid, or low on energy, or have other concerns, reach for your special stone. Hold it and remember the feeling you had when you helped energize the stone. It will help balance your energy and return you to a more centered, peaceful feeling.

Inner Connecting: Tiger Joy

Go to your special, quiet place for inner connecting and light a candle. Be sure there's not much air movement so the flame doesn't flicker and dance.

Sit quietly, focusing your attention on the candle flame. This will help you keep your mind still. If thoughts arise, just notice them and shift your attention back to the candle. Continue this for five to fifteen minutes or so. If you start feeling sleepy, close your eyes and stay in that same quiet space.

Essential Oil:

Lavender

- Put Lavender on your feet, wear as a perfume or cologne, or diffuse into the air. It helps balance the emotions, promotes spiritual consciousness, love, peace, and well-being, and helps reduce stress, tension, and fear of criticism. Historically it was used for just about everything.

More Steps to Tiger Joy

- Take time to nurture and heal yourself by letting your mind and body rest.

- Do something that makes your spirit soar. Is it an adventure or a thrilling, daring feat? Is it spending time in quiet contemplation, perhaps near a babbling brook or from a mountain vista? Whatever it is for you, do it often.

- When something happens that isn't according to your plan or desire (and it will), know that you'll be able to flow with it and be guided, possibly in another direction.

- Listen to classical music, soft jazz, or other easy, flowing music and feel the oneness as you flow with the music.

- Think of a time when you felt very much in the flow, at peace with yourself and the world around you. Where were you? What were you doing? You'll be able to feel the energy of that experience whenever you focus on it.

- Journal about your experiences of being fully present in the moment and about those that make your heart sing. Reread one or more of these from time to time. Set your intent to create that higher vibrational energy more frequently.

- Approach life with a positive "I can see this another way" attitude.

Healing Guide

Being and flowing with what is without resistance is empowering. What path are you on? If you aren't following a path of peace, love, hope, and inner joy, are you ready to change paths? You may feel like you're following a path, or you may be in the flow without a path. Whatever you're doing in this moment is right for you. Just keep listening to that tiger within, your inner guidance, and following it. It will lead you to an awareness of Beingness, Oneness, and Presence.

Coming
Home

EMPOWERMENT CAN BE DESCRIBED in many different ways. Each of them will lead you to the same place: using your inner knowing as a guide to inner peace and harmony. Throughout this book, I've used the term "empowerment" often, using stories, examples, and suggested activities for regaining or strengthening your power.

Empowerment is feeling the fear and doing it anyway. Empowerment is relying on that deep sense of knowing rather than doing what others say we should do or doing what we've always done before. Empowerment is believing that whatever choice we make is the right choice in this moment and being at peace with it. Empowerment is allowing others to follow their spiritual path without judgment and following our own path with peace and love in our hearts.

I've frequently referred to life as a journey with paths, roads, bridges, guides, and choices to make. Now, as our journey together comes to a close, I wish to leave you with a brief review to beingness, peace, and joy.

These nine paths to healing and empowerment are provided here as brief reminders of the journey you have undertaken.

1. **Release fears and limiting beliefs.**

   Let go of using past experiences, fears, and beliefs as excuses for the way your life is. Memories and fears from the past projected into the future keep you stuck in more of what you don't want. Rehashing your story with all of its drama only adds energy to staying stuck.

2. **Love and respect yourself and others.**

Treat yourself and others with compassion. Believe in yourself. Think and speak positively about yourself and others. Allow others to be who they are.

3. **Claim your power.**

Retrieve, retain, and use your inner power. If you feel power-less, change your perception of yourself and your situation. Make another choice using your inner knowing to guide you. Ask for help if you can't do it by yourself. Speak your truth.

4. **Follow your inner guidance.**

Practice techniques for getting in touch with your inner guidance. With practice you'll gain greater clarity and confidence.

5. **Balance body, mind, and spirit.**

When your body, mind, and spirit are in balance, you'll feel less stress, less dis-ease, and more peace.

6. **Connect with abundance.**

Abundance surrounds us and is always present. If you aren't experiencing it or feeling it, change your perception and your mind. Start looking for simple examples of abundance and express your gratitude for them. Abundance will begin flowing to and through you more easily.

The more you give gratitude, the more you have to be grateful for. When you express appreciation for what is, you increase that energy within you. You increase your awareness of it, expect it, feel it, and help create more of it. Make gratitude a way of life.

7. **Feel the oneness of All That Is .**

Love is the oneness and the essence of what is. You connect with everything and everyone from your heart. Release the need to understand. Give up comparing, judging, and deciding who's right and who's wrong. Staying in your mind keeps you feeling separate from All That Is .

8. Heal from your heart.

Connect with your heart-knowing and heart-remembering. Share from the heart. Show compassion for yourself and all things. Follow your passion.

9. Be at peace with what is in this moment.

Since you can see peace instead of this, why would you choose pain, suffering, and separation? Allow yourself and others to be, without resistance, complaints, negativity, and "shoulds."

Wishing you were somewhere else with someone else doing something else takes you away from the peace and joy of this moment. Let go of thinking you need to change, to be different, or to be or do more of this and less of that. There is nothing you need to do.

Be completely present in this moment. Your consciousness will naturally and easily connect with that place of beingness, peace, love, and joy within you. Be still, listen, and follow.

Consider placing this list of the nine paths where you'll see it daily. Choose one or two of the paths as your current focus for healing and empowerment. You can write them on an index card, carry it with you, and refer to it throughout the day as a reminder.

Be aware that these 9 Paths to Healing and Empowerment are offered only as guides or pointers to empowerment and inner peace. You may find them helpful for changing how you see yourself and the world around you.

However, neither memorizing the Empowerment Guides nor following all of the suggestions in the Action Guides at the end of the chapters will, in and of themselves, guarantee empowerment or happiness. They are merely tools to aid you on your journey.

You can spend lots of time or money on reading books like this one, meditating, attending seminars and classes, receiving special training, following spiritual teachers, and traveling to sacred sites. However, none of these activities will give you what you're seeking. They only point the way to the truth of beingness.

Are these things okay to do? Of course. Can they be helpful? Certainly. Honor where you are and what you feel guided to do now. As your awareness shifts, you'll be drawn to other activities or non-activity. That's okay too. Change paths, follow one of your own, be still, or just be.

> *Change paths, follow one of your own, be still, or just* **be.**

What is important? This question can be answered in many ways. It's whatever you think is important. It's what your search is about. You may be searching for your purpose in life.

Are you expecting to find something grand, exciting, or emotionally satisfying to do with your life? If so, you're still searching for answers in the world of form, outside of yourself. What you may think of as your life's purpose is usually something you're passionate about, a way to make a significant difference, or a desire to bring joy to yourself or others. You may have an intense yearning to discover this so that you can get on with what you came here to do.

What we do is not nearly as important as how we feel about who we are. It doesn't matter if we are religious, spiritual, agnostic, outgoing, withdrawn, healthy, ill, or "handicapped." How much money or education we have, what kind of work we do, the kind of car we drive, or whether we serve or are served do not affect the truth of our beingness.

If we believe we're here to overcome karma, challenges, or disappointments, or to learn lessons, then we'll draw more of those experiences to us. If we have a strong desire to be peaceful and joyful, then we're more likely to attract that into our lives.

What's not important or helpful for you? It's whatever you think. You choose.

The journey of healing and empowerment is a lot like being on a treasure hunt. You may have a list of many things or, perhaps, just one thing you want to find or do. Your search may take you all over the world.

You may go to Africa, Colorado, or California looking for gold. To find truth or your purpose in life, you may explore sacred texts from other religions and seek out spiritual teachers, sages, and gurus in the United States, China, India, or Tibet, and beyond.

Are you looking for that special tiger? You may choose to hunt for it in South America, Mexico, Africa, India, or Tibet. Have you gotten lost in the trees, nearly died from exhaustion and thirst, or almost drowned in raging waters only to discover that what you've been seeking isn't out there?

The **treasure** *is not hidden.*

Actually, no hunt is needed. The treasure is not hidden. It's always been in the same place inside you and all around you, available to all who are ready to claim it. As long as you think there's something more to search for, you'll continue your journey.

In fact, there is no journey except for the one in your mind. Since you have never really been separated from the source, no return journey is needed. Therefore, any path will get you where you want to be and no path will get you there also. However, thinking of a journey or a path may be a helpful guide, a comforting feeling, or simply a metaphor for life in a body. All paths lead to the same destination: truth, love, peace, beingness, and the oneness of All That Is.

If you're always at your spiritual home, how can you journey to your home? It would be like packing for a trip, sitting in the car in your driveway with all of your stuff, and trying to figure out what to do and which way to go to get home.

Think of it like a game, knowing you're not really going anywhere, but still pretending you are. You'll realize the game is just a game and isn't real. Eventually you'll get tired of sitting in your driveway and will end the game, and go inside.

No one can give you a map that shows all the places along your journey, and ensures you'll arrive where you wanted to be and at the time you wanted to arrive. Your mind can let go of the belief that you are somewhere else without a road map looking for your true home and your true self. Because your mind and your ego find that difficult to accept, you may find it helpful to use tools, guides, and paths to point the way.

It is discovering that the tiger within has always been there, fully awake.

However, the journey of healing and empowerment doesn't have to be a long process. Actually it's much easier than you may think. Stop thinking you're far away and enjoy being at home surrounded by peace and joy. Since you're already home and have always been one with the source, the shift in awareness can happen now. Truly, it can only happen now, in this moment.

What is your purpose? It is discovering the truth of who you are. It is a journey of the heart or no journey at all. It's ending the search. It is discovering that the tiger within has always been there, fully awake.

Beyond the
Words

ULTIMATELY THE TRUTH OF KNOWING who you are at a deeper level, discovering the tiger within, is beyond any words. Healing, empowerment, peace, and love are really more than any definition or verbal description can convey.

The truth is more about a feeling, a deeper connection or an inner sense of what is. When we stop resisting what is, when our minds slow down enough so that the words stop ...that's peace or beingness.

The truth can be found in allowing "it" to be: yourself, others, the world around you. It's when you allow what is to just be, without judging it or trying to change it into something other than that. It's who you are before you think about who you are and before you try to be different.

Relax, listen, flow, and be as you connect with the essence of the message beyond the words. Truth is the nothingness out of which everything flows and is. It's what is, before the words, before the thoughts, before the emotions.

Truth is not about the past or the future. It's about beingness in this moment. That's All That Is. It's really that simple. Be at peace or Oneness with what is, with yourself, and with your creations. Smile, breathe, and be joyful.

Namaste.

Truth is the **nothingness** *out of which everything flows and is.*

Taking Your Tiger By the Tail

Following the Steps on Your Path

NOW IS THE TIME to consider all that you've read and experienced. Spend some time quietly reflecting on what will help your life feel more peaceful. Ask for guidance about how you want to feel and be while coming from a place of empowerment. Listen to your inner tiger for greater clarity and insight.

What will you focus on? What will you do to shift away from old, energy-draining patterns? Complete and use the guide (outline) below to assist you in taking steps toward bringing more peace and joy into your life and into your beingness.

Then review the guide first thing in the morning and before going to bed at night. While you may not always be aware of the more subtle shifts in your responses and life occurrences on a daily basis, know that they are taking place.

If something comes up that draws you away from the intentions you wrote in your personal guide, just regroup as soon as you can and continue on. At the end of each week, go back to the beginning of the week, and see what changes you notice. At the end of each month, you will see some significant differences.

Make adjustments to the steps you've outlined in the Taking My Tiger by the Tail Guide according to what feels right and useful to you. Are you ready to change some of the steps, add steps, or move on to another area? When you start on a new area, continue to strengthen yourself and reinforce the shifts you've made in the previous areas.

Now that you have the basic idea, go to the next page and begin to focus on the steps you can commit to taking. (Hint: Make copies of the Taking My Tiger by the Tail Guide so that you can use it for following your steps on several different paths. You have my permission to copy the guide specified above for this purpose only.)

Taking My
Tiger by the Tail
Guide

Connect with your inner tiger, ask for guidance about the path you choose to focus on, and complete each step according to what feels right to you. Select ideas and activities from the book or create your own. Use this as a daily guide for claiming your power.

1. Which of the nine paths are you going to follow now?

   _____

2. List one or two points related to the Empowerment Guide that support you on the path and have meaning for you.

   _____

   _____

3. Now choose some activities that you feel are helpful to you. List or describe briefly below. Adding a page number from the book may be helpful.

Affirmation:

_____

_____

Energy Technique:

_____

_____

Inner Connecting:

_____

_____

Essential Oils:

_____

_____

4. What additional steps do you feel guided to focus on? Make some of these very specific to feeling peace in your life situation. Consider how you can respond differently or see the person or situation in a more positive way.

_____

_____

_____

_____

_____

_____

I am committed to claiming my power and finding peace in my life.

_____

Signature   Date

Taking My
Tiger by the Tail
Review

AT THE END OF EACH WEEK and before moving to another path, review your progress on your chosen path. Complete each of the statements below.

1. What I have discovered about myself is:

_____

_____

2. What makes me feel peaceful about my focus and follow through on this path is:

_____

_____

3. I am grateful for:

_____

_____

4. I deserve:

_____

_____

5. I choose to recognize and reward myself for:

_____

_____

_____

_____

_____

Signature   Date

Suggested Readings and Resources

Books

20,000 Dreams by Mary Summer Rain (Thunder Bay Press, 2006)

The Artist's Way by Julia Cameron (The Putnam Publishing Group, 1992)

A Course in Miracles (Public Domain)

Emptiness Dancing by Adyashanti (Sounds True, 2006)

Energy Medicine by Donna Eden (Tarcher/Putnam, 1998)

The Eye of the I by David R. Hawkins, M.D., Ph.D (Veritas Publishing, 2001)

Joy's Way by W. Brugh Joy, M.D. (Tarcher/Putnam, 1979)

A New Earth by Eckhart Tolle (Penguin Group, 2005)

Reference Guide for Essential Oils by Connie and Alan Higley (Abundant Health, revised 2002)

The Seven Spiritual Laws of Success by Deepak Chopra, M.D. (Amber-Allen Publishing and New World Library, 1993)

There's A Spiritual Solution to Every Problem by Wayne W. Dyer (HarperCollins Publishers, 2001)

Wake Up Inspired by Marion Baker (New Story Press, 2006)

Why Your Life Sucks by Alan Cohen (Bantam Dell, 2005)

You Can Heal Your Life by Louise Hay (Hay House, 1984)

Your Body Speaks Your Mind by Deb Shapiro (Sounds True, 2006)

Additional Energy Healing Resources

www.healingtouchinternational.org

www.healingtouchprogram.com

Additional Options for Growth and Exploration

More Support for Continuing on Your Path

This book is just one tool for you to use on your journey to wholeness, healing, and empowerment. Reading a book does not replace other options of working individually with a healing professional, meeting in small, nurturing support groups, or getting additional training through classes and workshops. If you are looking for more ways to shift your consciousness and let go of old patterns, we offer continuing support through a wide variety of other resources and opportunities. We at Heartsong Healing are passionate about providing what it takes to help you use your power for self-healing and helping others heal.

Circles of Joy

"Circles of Joy" will help you raise your energetic vibration and spread joy to others and to the world around you. As one of a small group of caring individuals, ready to find and awaken the joy that is already deep inside, you'll continue your journey through guided activities and sharing experiences. For more information or to register for "Circles of Joy," go to our website at www.awakeningthetigerwithin.com or send us an e-mail at awakenthetiger@heartsonghealing.net.

Tiger Talk Wisdom Circles

"Tiger Talk Wisdom Circles" explore and teach, in a small-group format, how you can look at challenging experiences with new eyes and a new approach. We address real-life situations, suggest specific techniques and ideas, and share individual and group insights. Check out our website to sign up for our "Tiger Talk Wisdom Circles" or e-mail us. (See links above.)

Website Help and Information

Join our growing list of users at www.awakeningthetigerwithin.com for motivating stories, free materials, and other resources to assist you on your journey. Be sure to leave us your contact information so you can begin receiving our newsletter and other special offers.

Classes and Workshops

Workshops based on *Awakening the Tiger Within: 9 Paths to Healing and Empowerment* are offered as a series of three or can be taken individually either onsite or through teleclasses. For more details or for a complete list of workshops and classes, see our website.

One-on-One Energy Healing Sessions

One-on-one healing sessions are individualized and intuitively guided. We emphasize meeting your needs, focusing on the "highest good" for maximum benefit. Individual sessions are done onsite or through distance healing.

Contact Joy by e-mail at: awakenthetiger@heartsonghealing.net to get more information or to schedule.

Client Comments:

After one visit to see Joy, the severe pain I had been in for about ten years was significantly reduced. After a couple more sessions, the pain was almost totally gone; I have been able to resume all of my normal activities; I no longer need the surgery the doctors recommended.
— Timothy Bandrowsky, D.D.S., Maxillofacial Surgeon

"Joy helps reinforce that I'm okay and that I can move forward. I know it, but being able to overcome past conditioning and experiences is challenging. She helps me replace old beliefs and release old emotional patterns."
— Linda Bosserman, Business Owner

I experience wonderful, great energy shifts every time. It's as if we're able to shift energy in places I hadn't been able to reach with other healers. Transformational! It's easy to trust Joy's work is for the highest good."
— Rev. Rosemary Bredeson, Spiritual Counselor

Speaking Engagements

Joy focuses her presentations on helping others claim their true power by connecting with the wisdom of the Tiger within. She is available to inspire, and teach and share stories, insights, and techniques from successes with both clients and her own healing journey in a variety of large- and small-group forums. Joy will tailor her presentation to meet the needs of your group. Check out our website and send us an e-mail with your specific request and questions.

Share Your Stories and Comments

We'd love to hear from you! How has this book and working with the ideas and follow-up suggestions inspired you or changed your life? What new perspectives and insights have you gained? Tell us how we can help as you continue on your path. Submit your stories, thoughts, and feedback on the book through the e-mail link available on the website.

Contact Information

www.awakeningthetigerwithin.com
Email: awakenthetiger@heartsonghealing.net

To Order Copies of this Book

www.awakeningthetigerwithin.com
Email: awakenthetiger@heartsonghealing.net

Inquire about volume or special discounts available.

About the Author

Joy Heartsong's healing journey took a new path after a personal health crisis led to her retirement from a 25-year career as a teacher and public school administrator. In the successful quest to regain her health, Joy discovered the power of healing touch and energy healing which subsequently led her to a career rebirth in the healing arts. As a Certified Healing Touch Practitioner and Biofield Energy Therapist, she has helped hundreds of clients achieve greater balance in body, mind, and spirit.

In her latest work, *Awakening the Tiger Within,* Joy describes *9 Paths to Healing and Empowerment.* The techniques Joy recommends in this book have been developed through her extensive experience helping others access their own inner power for both physical and personal healing.

Joy currently lives and works in beautiful Colorado Springs, Colorado and remains dedicated to her private practice even as the demand for her classes, workshops, and speaking engagements grows.

Printed in the United States
99171LV00004B/334-351/A

9 780979 981807